The Reproductive Industry

Critical Perspectives on Psychology of Sexuality, Gender, and Queer Studies

Mission Statement

The series seeks to publish scholarship that engages critically with the social and political uses of psychological knowledge, and with transformative paradigms that address obstacles to change. The series is open to a wide range of approaches that may be classified as "psychological," including manuscript proposals that focus on well-being, subjectivities, clinical practice, discourse, and their intersections.

Books in Series

The Reproductive Industry: Intimate Experiences and Global Processes, edited by Vera Mackie, Nicola J. Marks, and Sarah Ferber
The Psychic Life of Racism in Gay Men's Communities, edited by Damien W. Riggs

The Reproductive Industry

Intimate Experiences and Global Processes

Edited by
Vera Mackie, Nicola J. Marks,
and Sarah Ferber

LEXINGTON BOOKS
Lanham • Boulder • New York • London

Published by Lexington Books
An imprint of The Rowman & Littlefield Publishing Group, Inc.
4501 Forbes Boulevard, Suite 200, Lanham, Maryland 20706
www.rowman.com

6 Tinworth Street, London SE11 5AL, United Kingdom

British Library Cataloguing in Publication Information Available

Library of Congress Cataloging-in-Publication Data

ISBN 978-1-4985-7065-7 (cloth)
ISBN 978-1-4985-7066-4 (electronic)

Contents

Acknowledgments

This edited collection is the outcome of a major research project funded by Australian Research Council Discovery Project DP150101081 and led by the volume's editors Sarah Ferber, Vera Mackie, and Nicola J. Marks.

A workshop funded by the Academy of the Social Sciences in Australia and the University of Wollongong allowed us to invite the leading international scholars in the field, as well as emerging scholars, and to provide our authors with expert feedback on their draft chapters. Our research associate, Robyn Morris, provided support throughout the project and assisted with convening the workshop. Samson Soulsby provided invaluable editorial assistance in preparing the final manuscript. Alexander Brown prepared the index.

We would like to express our sincere thanks to Kasey Beduhn and her staff from Lexington Books for their ongoing support, and the editorial board of the Critical Perspectives on the Psychology of Sexuality, Gender and Queer Studies book series for their encouragement.

Introduction

The Body and the Globe

Vera Mackie, Nicola J. Marks, and Sarah Ferber

Stories of assisted reproduction from around the world are ubiquitous in the mass media.[1] In March 2013, a Chinese couple, Shen Jie and Liu Xi, were killed in a car crash, five days before they were due to have embryos implanted through in vitro fertilization (IVF). After a legal battle, both sets of parents of the deceased couple were able to access the frozen embryos stored in a hospital in Nanjing. Through a surrogacy agency, two embryos were implanted into the womb of a Lao woman who traveled to China on a tourist visa and gave birth to a baby boy, four years after the death of the intended parents. The grandparents are now raising the child (Ramzy 2018).

Chen Huang, a single woman from the People's Republic of China, researched sperm donation and IVF on the internet and decided to go to Australia for treatment, a place where she had previously studied. Her gynecologist in Sydney speaks Chinese, and increasingly sees clients who travel to Australia for treatment. Although the one-child policy in China was relaxed in 2016, as a single woman, Chen did not have access to sperm donation or IVF. The rise of an affluent middle class in China in the twenty-first century has seen them travel overseas as international students or on shorter trips as tourists. These forces help to explain how and why Chen was able to travel to Australia to choose a sperm donor, undergo IVF, and eventually bear a child (SBS News 2017). Meanwhile poorer women in Chinese villages are acting as gestational surrogates for more wealthy Chinese couples (Chen 2017).

Natalie Lovett was 46 and childless when she flew from Australia to the United States to create a baby. She was treated at a San Diego fertility clinic and gave birth to a daughter. She was then faced with the decision of what to do with the extra embryos stored in the clinic. Eventually she decided to create a new form of family. She offered her embryos to other intending parents, on the understanding that the offspring would form part of an extended family for her daughter, Lexie. The embryos have been donated to single childless women, same-sex couples, and heterosexual couples, and Lexie now has several "diblings" (donor siblings) to whom she is genetically related (ABC 2015; Caines 2017; Lovett 2017).

Stories of celebrities' use of assisted reproduction (Ottolenghi 2014) contrast with those of the exploitation of gestational surrogate mothers and of abandoned babies (Murdoch 2017). Reproduction increasingly involves various forms of border crossing. The most intimate, embodied elements of biological reproduction are embedded in global processes. This is why this book refers to "intimate experiences and global processes."[2]

While the aforementioned stories attest to the formation of new families in previously unthinkable ways, other stories highlight the fragility of these processes. A common side effect of disasters which disrupt power supplies is a threat to the viability of frozen gametes and embryos. After the Fukushima tsunami, earthquake and nuclear disaster in Japan in March 2011, gynecologists reported "several sad and unfortunate consequences" of the earthquake.

> Twelve clinics lost at least one embryo. Two reports described loss of embryos with spilled culture medium in the incubator. In one case the embryologist dropped an embryo on the floor at the time of transfer when the earth tremor suddenly started. A similar loss of an embryo was reported during a vitrification procedure. Three clinics reported that prolonged power failure caused possible deterioration of embryos in incubators. Of 78 clinics experiencing unexpected power cuts, 65 had been equipped in advance with some equipment for emergency power supply backup. However, prolonged power failure at the disaster resulted in other difficulties, including unstable voltage supply and unexpected fuel shortage for generators. (Ishihara and Yoshimura 2011, 8)

Disasters also highlight the fragility of the relationships between different parties to surrogacy arrangements. On April 25, 2015, an earthquake struck Kathmandu, the capital of Nepal. Approximately 9,000 people died and many thousands were injured or displaced (Rafferty n.d.). Among those affected were Israeli gay couples waiting to return home with babies recently born to gestational mothers. Israel was quick to send in military aircraft to evacuate the fathers and twenty-six babies (Lewis 2015; Eglash 2015). Some commentators, though, noted the lack of any mention of the gestational mothers who were left behind (Green 2015). Eventually, some of the women were also evacuated to Israel where they could remain until they gave birth (Robertson 2015). In 2018, people took to the streets in Tel Aviv after gay men were again excluded from surrogacy access in new legislation in Israel (Amichai 2018). Fragility in the processes of assisted reproduction is in some ways the hallmark of IVF. The fragility of these processes arises as a result of reliance on technology and is embedded in the context of inequalities in global geography and politics. Globalized assisted reproduction has provided greater opportunities for some people to reproduce, but on terms which implicate them and others in a chain of contingencies.

The first babies conceived through IVF (then popularly known as "test tube babies")[3] were born in 1978 in the United Kingdom and in India (Franklin 1995; Bharadwaj 2002). They were soon followed by births in such places as Australia in 1980, the United States in 1981, France, Sweden, Israel, Finland, Germany, the Netherlands, Czech Republic, Canada, Greece, and Austria each in 1982, and Japan, Belgium, Denmark, and Singapore in 1983. This area of research initially had difficulty obtaining funding and achieving successful pregnancies and births. Four decades later, assisted reproduction is a global industry, present in many, though not all, countries (Inhorn and Patrizio 2015). In many ways IVF and assisted reproductive technologies (ARTs) have become commonplace and normalized because they are seen to help people have the families they desire (Thompson 2005; Franklin 2013b). In other ways assisted reproduction remains controversial because the numbers of "take-home" babies per IVF cycle remain lower than what "miracle baby" media stories or IVF clinics' advertisements might suggest (Spar 2006).

Sperm, eggs, and the embryos created through these technologies can be bought and sold for varying sums of money, while others are paid to gestate babies on behalf of commissioning parents. These transactions take place across national borders, often through the mediation of agents, and can be exploitative (Gürtin and Inhorn 2011; Pande 2016). Babies born following IVF and surrogacy arrangements can remain stuck in countries due to complex configurations of local and international family laws. There may be difficulties in registering babies in the home country of the commissioning parents, with some children left stateless and illegitimate (van Wichelen in this volume; Mackie 2013, 2014a).

People have used these technologies to create diverse family forms, including gay, lesbian, and transgender parenthood and complex configurations of genetic, gestational, and social parenthood (as exemplified in Natalie Lovett's story above; see also Mamo 2007; Luce 2010; Riggs in this volume; Keaney in this volume). There have been calls to rethink these ways of doing reproduction or at least to regulate them more effectively (Whittaker 2011; Daniels and Heidt-Forsythe 2012; Pande 2014).

After more than forty years of assisted reproduction since IVF, it seems timely to reflect on the global dimensions of IVF and the associated assisted reproductive technologies. In this collection, we think of these technologies as ways of reproducing kin, families, and genetic heritage. These technologies are also, though, involved in the reproduction—and sometimes reconfiguration—of norms, cultures, and ways of thinking and doing (Franklin 1997, 2013a, 2013b). In this collection, our contributors explore how reproductive technologies, like other technologies, have shaped and been shaped by social and cultural factors across time and across the globe.

While we are interested in global processes, we do not see globalization as a one-way, all-encompassing and unstoppable force. Rather, we think of globalization as made up of multiple locally situated processes, which move in multiple directions (Mackie and Stevens 2009; Anderson 2014), as can be seen in the vignettes above. Thus, there is a focus on case study chapters which pay attention to local spatial, historical, and cultural situations while revealing the dynamics of global processes.

There is a complex interaction between the local and the global. Discussion of family and reproduction is often focused on discourses of the national. Governments attempt to manage their populations in various ways, in what Foucault has referred to as "biopolitics" (1978, 2008; Rabinow and Rose 2006). Franklin and Inhorn (2016) describe "repronationalism", which refers not to the passive way in which IVF is shaped by local circumstances, but the active ways in which the governance of IVF is used to shape national politics, morality, foreign policy, and the economy. Franklin (in this volume) argues that

> official national policies about IVF and other reproductive technologies concern not only fertility and demography, or medical ethics, but the basic guiding principles toward health and welfare systems, and even the core definition of the social contract linking citizens to the state.

There is evidence of distinctive discourses of repronationalism in the case study chapters on the United Kingdom, India, and Thailand (Franklin in this volume; Mohanka in this volume; Whittaker in this volume; on repronationalism in Japan, see Mackie 2009, 2013, 2014a, 2014b). Cultural representations are also important in imagining which kinds of families are seen as belonging to the nation (Whittaker in this volume; Mackie 2018).

Governments try to regulate reproduction in various ways. They may prohibit the use of certain forms of assisted reproduction. They may place conditions on the use of assisted reproduction, such as restricting the use of these technologies to married couples in heteronormative relationships, or by prohibiting their use by non-nationals. Some states in federal systems may facilitate the use of assisted reproduction, such as the US states of Nevada and California, which regulate surrogacy contracts and the issue of birth certificates. Other governments choose not to regulate—such as Japan, which has no legislative regulation, but only guidelines issued by the Japan Society of Obstetricians and Gynecologists. Failure to regulate, however, is also a form of regulation, allowing various practices to take place, as was the case in India and Thailand until recently. These gaps in regulation between different nation-states or between different states in federal systems are one of the reasons for choices to cross borders in search of reproductive services.

The chapters in this volume critically explore how IVF and other assisted reproductive technologies have circulated (or not) around the globe; what is being produced and reproduced through processes such as IVF, fertility preservation, gamete commercialization, or surrogacy; how reproductive technologies can be situated historically, nationally, locally, transnationally, geographically, and culturally; the meanings of reproductive technologies in culture and in practice; and the ways in which culture, practices, regulations, norms, families, and kinship ties may be reinforced or challenged through the use of assisted reproduction.

This volume contributes to the literature arguing for the importance of exploring ARTs beyond the Global North (Knecht et al. 2012; Sarojini and Marwah 2015; Franklin and Inhorn 2016; Bärnreuther 2016; Rozée and Unisa 2016) with several chapters focusing on the Asia-Pacific region. Case study chapters draw on a diverse range of approaches and theories (including insights from history, psychology, law, ethnography, science and technology studies, cultural studies, literary studies, postcolonial studies, gender and sexuality studies, queer theory, and critical race and whiteness studies) to explore the complex cultural and historical situatedness of global IVF and ARTs.

The first set of chapters offers historical analyses of factors shaping IVF and ARTs. Sarah Franklin explores the changing contexts in which IVF developed in the United Kingdom, and how the move from the early post–Second World War welfare state to Margaret Thatcher's (1925–2013) "enterprise culture" influenced this technology. Whereas the 1970s National Health Service (NHS) under Labour Party governments had been oriented toward an inclusive ethos of care and repair, the Thatcherite NHS of the 1980s was modeled on a social contract drawn from the free market—where competition was prized as a moral and financial good. The emergence of IVF in the United Kingdom was not merely a consequence of these trends, but helped to shape and drive major shifts in the ways in/fertility, technology, governance, and welfare were defined as the twentieth century came to a close.

Vasudha Mohanka revisits and updates the social, political, and cultural contexts of IVF in India, a key site for global IVF until the enactment of the Surrogacy Regulation Bill in December 2018.[4] In the past few years, she argues, the emphasis on restricting the use of reproductive services like IVF and surrogacy to particular kinds of groups and families reflects the state's role in creating and encouraging particular types of familial and kinship arrangements and disregarding others. These repronational histories and choreographies (Thompson 2005) reveal the role of different actors and institutions—from religion and media, to the state and family—which influence the use of and access to technologies such as IVF in particular social, political, economic, and cultural contexts.

Jane Adams provides a historical analysis of debates on artificial insemination by donor (AID) in New Zealand, including developments in family law, human rights law, and responsiveness to Māori perspectives. In mid-twentieth-century New Zealand, AI was seen as a secretive, shameful practice. Through its legal association with adultery and divorce, it was perceived that it could potentially destroy families. By the 1980s, AI had become a more established medical practice, and politicians responded to it positively, acknowledging its ability to allow infertile married couples to become parents—and in doing so, to possibly "save" troubled marriages. Donor secrecy was still assumed, however, as the two-parent heterosexual family remained the ideal, and concurrent developments in adoption and homosexual law reform were not considered. Within ten years, donor openness in ART—promoted by a resurgence in Māori culture, human rights developments, open adoption practices, egg donation programs, and greater visibility of same-sex couples as parents—had become the new norm.[5] What had once been a marital secret for heterosexual parents within a nuclear family was now a more open practice accessible to a far wider range of adults, and subject to official record-keeping and regulation. While the first babies conceived through IVF generally used the gametes of the intending parents, sperm donation allowed a greater number of couples to access assisted reproduction (see also Adams 2016).

The next set of chapters focuses on perspectives from important stakeholders in IVF who are sometimes missing from mainstream narratives. Damien Riggs builds on his experience as a psychotherapist to explore the complexities of discussing fertility preservation options with transgender youth. In these discussions, argues Riggs, there is often a slippage between "wanting to have a child" and "fertility." This slippage positions transgender people's potential desire to become parents within a pronatalist logic where only genetic reproduction is valued. This ignores other pathways to parenthood available to transgender people, such as permanent foster care in Australia, adoption in other countries (given low adoption rates in Australia), and a partner carrying a child conceived from donor gametes. From an ethical position, he argues that advocating that transgender people seek a place within the norm of genetic reproduction is likely to produce distress for those for whom the costs of fertility preservation can be prohibitive. Storage fees—until such time as the individual decides to use or dispose of frozen gametes—are not inconsiderable, and well beyond the means of many transgender people in the context of multiple other expenses for gender reassignment surgery or hormone treatments, which may only be supported by private health insurance.

Jaya Keaney draws on in-depth interviews with queer parents to explore how concepts of "race" are reconfigured through third-party provision of gametes. Where past Anglophone literature, public culture, and clinical practice around assisted reproduction has centered the white, heterosexual, middle-class infertile couple,[6] Keaney argues that the queer multiracial family is emerging as a powerful emblem of the drastic changes in the landscape of contemporary kinship. The inequality of global formations of racialization is woven into the fabric of fertility markets, yet "race" in gamete selection is overwhelmingly cast as a benign liberal consumer choice (Cooper and Waldby 2014, 64–65; Schurr 2017, 1–2). She presents the queer multiracial family figuration in the hope that it might offer imaginative resources for thinking critically about how the concept of "race" is always delineated, encountered, and rearranged by the reproductive arrangements that produce it.

Robyn Morris explores patient perspectives on IVF through a literary analysis of Australian memoirs concerning IVF and assisted reproduction. Personal narratives provide insights into the embodied and subjective dimensions of undergoing IVF treatment. Some narratives focus on "successful" IVF procedures which result in the birth of a child, while others focus on those who are not able to have children after years of procedures and who therefore must reorient their life goals. These memoirs also reveal how individuals come to terms with the realities of the low success rates of IVF procedures, contrary to often triumphalist narratives of medical breakthroughs.

A final set of chapters places the global dimensions of IVF at the center of analysis. Sonja van Wichelen explores the regulation of global surrogacy from a legal perspective. The Hague Conference on Private International Law (HCCH) is an intergovernmental organization responsible for the regulation of private matters across different jurisdictions. Over the years, it has adopted numerous conventions which aim to harmonize conflict of law situations. The status of children has been a primary focus. Existing conventions in this area include those on child abduction, child maintenance obligations, and intercountry adoption. There has been discussion of whether there needs to be an international convention on cross-border surrogacy. Van Wichelen poses the following question: when genetics—or biology—is allowed to travel across borders, while social, intentional, or de facto relations cannot, how can we think about regulating the private in the broader context of the social and the global? In the absence of an international convention on cross-border surrogacy, some invoke the United Nations Convention on the Rights of the Child (1989), which states that when making decisions about children "the interests of the child shall be a primary consideration" (Article 3). Every child has the "right to know and be cared for by his or her parents" (Article 17: 1), the "right to identity," and the right to a nationality (Article 8) (Wade 2017; Gerber and O'Byrne 2016).

Andrea Whittaker analyzes Thai media reporting of some controversial surrogacy cases—the "Baby Gammy" case and the Japanese man, Shigeta Mitsutoki, who fathered over a dozen children through surrogacy. Each of these cases involved a non-Thai father with Thai women as gestational mothers. The public debate over surrogacy evoked an image of Thai women's bodies as symbolic boundaries of the nation being breached by foreign forces, echoing earlier controversies about the transnational sex work industry. The international controversies on cross-border surrogacy prompted the government to enact the Protection for Children Born Through Assisted Reproductive Technologies Act. This Act enforced the ban on commercial surrogacy and commercial ovum donation and disallowed intermediaries or brokers for surrogacy arrangements. It restricted the eligibility for surrogacy to heterosexual couples (at least one of whom must be Thai) who have been married for at least two years. In addition, it requires the women who gestate to be female relatives of the couples requesting surrogacy.

In the concluding chapter, Marks, Mackie, and Ferber analyze factors shaping reproductive mobilities in the Asia-Pacific region. This chapter brings together the book's themes of the enmeshment of globalization and the growth of the assisted reproduction industry. The chapter illustrates these processes by tracing reproductive mobilities to and from the nodes of Japan, Australia, and the French Pacific. Each of these nodes is associated with particular, at times intersecting, routes to destinations where reproductive services are available. IVF and ARTs are tightly woven into complex movements—as well as restrictions and transformations—affecting scientists, techniques, and scientific publications; biological material (eggs, sperm, embryos); bodies (providers of gametes, commissioning parents, gestational mothers, infertile couples, babies); capital; and regulatory discourses and cultural norms. Factors associated with the modes and routes of reproductive travel include the existence or lack of regulation, gaps between regulatory regimes in different places, gaps between the availability of particular reproductive medical services in different places, the promotion of medical travel and reproductive travel in particular local sites, economic inequality, linguistic or cultural connectedness, historical connections, diasporic connections, former colonial relationships, and geographical proximity. The routes of reproductive travel are not predictable or obvious, but need to be tracked through the kinds of micro-level case studies carried out in this volume.

NOTES

1. This edited collection is the outcome of a major research project funded by Australian Research Council Discovery Project DP150101081 and led by the volume's editors Sarah Ferber, Vera Mackie, and Nicola J. Marks. We would also like to acknowledge the work of Robyn Morris, research associate on the project. A workshop funded by the Academy of the Social Sciences in Australia and the University of Wollongong allowed us to invite the leading international scholars in the field, as well as emerging scholars, and to provide our authors with expert feedback on their draft chapters.

2. On the global dimensions of IVF and ARTS, see also Ferber, Mackie, and Marks (in press).

3. The fertilization actually took place in a petri dish rather than a test tube.

4. The Surrogacy Regulation Bill 2016 (Government of India 2018) was passed by the Lok Sabha (Lower House of Parliament) in December 2018 (Singh 2019). The Bill was initially approved by the Cabinet in August 2016. It was introduced in the Lower House in November 2016 and was then referred to a parliamentary standing committee on health and family welfare in January 2017 (Dey 2019; Banghra 2019; for further details see Mohanka in this volume).

5. Māori families had long practiced forms of adoption within their extended families and communities and found the secrecy associated with "closed" adoption and AID to be anathema. Part of the law reforms were aimed at addressing these concerns. On adoption and the use of ARTs in the French Pacific, see Marks (2017).

6. While it is the white, middle-class heterosexual couple which is centered in discourses of reproduction in Anglophone societies, each nation displays distinctive discourses of repronationalism which privilege particular classes and ethnicities, as can be seen in several of our case study chapters (Mohanka in this volume; Whittaker in this volume).

WORKS CITED

ABC. 2015. "Lexie's Village." *Australian Story*, September 29. http://www.abc.net.au/austory/lexies-village/7202730 (Last accessed June 29, 2018).

Adams, Jane. 2016. "'The Coital Factor': Medico-Legal Approaches towards Sexual Incapacity and Infertile Marriages in Mid-Twentieth Century New Zealand." *New Zealand Journal of History* 50 (1): 88–108.

Amichai, Rami. 2018. "Israel's LGBT Community Protests for Fathers' Surrogacy Rights." *Reuters*, July 22. https://www.reuters.com/article/us-israel-lgbt-protest/israels-lgbt-community-protests-for-fathers-surrogacy-rights-idUSKBN1KC0B3 (Last accessed July 26, 2018).

Anderson, Warwick. 2014. "Making Global Health History: The Postcolonial Worldliness of Biomedicine." *Social History of Medicine* 27 (2): 372–84.

Bärnreuther, Sandra. 2016. "Innovations 'Out of Place': Controversies Over IVF Beginnings in India between 1978 and 2005." *Medical Anthropology* 35 (1): 73–89.

Bhangra, Kulraj Singh. 2019. "India's Lower House Passes Bill Banning Commercial Surrogacy." *Bionews* 982 (January 14). Available at https://www.bionews.org.uk/page_140769 (Last accessed February 2, 2019).

Bharadwaj, Aditya. 2002. "Conception Politics: Medical Egos, Media Spotlights, and the Contest over Test Tube Firsts in India." In *Infertility Around the Globe: New Thinking on Childlessness, Gender, and Reproductive Technologies*, edited by Marcia Inhorn and Frank Van Balen, 315–33. Berkeley: University of California Press.

Caines, Kimberley. 2017. "Natalie Lovett Shared 24 Embryos to Create a Fraternal Village." *News.Com*, October 10. https://www.news.com.au/lifestyle/parenting/pregnancy/natalie-lovett-shared-24-embryos-to-create-a-fraternal-village/news-story/087c0fba705a2d5fe7b3723eea85cb4c (Last accessed September 30, 2018).

Chen, Stephen. 2017. "Surrogate Motherhood Becomes a Family Industry in Poor Chinese Villages." *South China Morning Post*, December 31. https://www.scmp.com/news/china/society/article/2126286/surrogate-motherhood-becomes-family-industry-poor-chinese (Last accessed September 30, 2018).

Cooper, Melinda and Catherine Waldby. 2014. *Clinical Labor: Tissue Donors and Research Subjects in the Global Bioeconomy*. Durham: Duke University Press.

Daniels, Cynthia R. and Erin Heidt-Forsythe. 2012. "Gendered Eugenics and the Problematic of Free Market Reproductive Technologies: Sperm and Egg Donation in the United States." *Signs: Journal of Women in Culture and Society* 37 (3): 719–47.

Dasgupta, Sayantani and Shamita Das Dasgupta, eds. 2014. *Globalization and Transnational Surrogacy in India: Outsourcing Life*. Lanham, MD: Lexington Books.

Dey, Sushmi. 2018. "Lok Sabha Clears Bill Banning Commercial Surrogacy." *Times of India*, December 20. Available at https://timesofindia.indiatimes.com/india/lok-sabha-passes-surrogacy-regulation-bill-2016-which-bans-commercial-surrogacy/articleshow/67165408.cms (Last accessed February 2, 2019).

Eglash, Ruth. 2015. "Among Nepal's Earthquake Survivors: Israeli Gays and their Surrogate Babies." *Washington Post*, April 30. https://www.washingtonpost.com/world/how-an-earthquake-highlighted-the-plight-of-israeli-gays-and-their-surrogate-babies/2015/04/29/419d60e8-ecf0-11e4-8050-839e9234b303_story.html?noredirect=on&utm_term=.ad8d7373b6d5 (Last accessed September 29, 2018).

Ferber, Sarah, Nicola J. Marks, and Vera Mackie. in press. *IVF and Assisted Reproduction: A Global History*. London: Palgrave Macmillan.

Foucault, Michel. 1978. *The History of Sexuality, Volume 1: The Will to Knowledge*. Translated by Robert Hurley. Harmondsworth: Penguin.

———. 2008. *The Birth of Biopolitics: Lectures at the Collège de France, 1978–79*. edited by Michel Senellart, translated by Graham Burchell. London: Palgrave Macmillan.

Franklin, Sarah. 1995. "Postmodern Procreation: A Cultural Account of Assisted Reproduction." In *Conceiving the New World Order: The Global Politics of Reproduction,* edited by Faye D. Ginsburg and Rayna Rapp, 323–45. California: University of California Press.

———. 1997. *Embodied Progress: A Cultural Account of Assisted Conception*. London: Routledge.

———. 2013a. *Biological Relatives: IVF, Stem Cells, and the Future of Kinship*. Durham: Duke University Press.

———. 2013b. "Conception through a Looking Glass: The Paradox of IVF." *Reproductive BioMedicine Online* 27 (6): 747–55.

———. 2016. "Changing Global Fertilities: A Third Demographic Transition." *ReproSoc*, May 16. http://www.reprosoc.com/blog/2016/11/30/changing-global-fertilities-a-third-demographic-transition.

Franklin, Sarah and Marcia Inhorn, eds. 2016. "Symposium: IVF – Global Histories." *Reproductive Biomedicine & Society Online* 2: 1–136.

Gerber, Paula and Katie O'Byrne. 2016. "Souls in the House of Tomorrow: The Rights of Children Born via Surrogacy." In *Surrogacy, Law and Human Rights*, edited by Paula Gerber and Katie O'Byrne, 81–112. Farnham: Ashgate.

Government of India. 2018. The Surrogacy Regulation Bill, Bill No 257-C of 2016, Passed by Lok Sabha on December 19, 2018.

Green, Alon-Lee. 2015. "Where Is the Concern for the Surrogate Mothers in Nepal?" April 27. https://www.haaretz.com/opinion/.premium-what-about-the-surrogates-in-nepal-1.5355284 (Last accessed September 29, 2018).

Gürtin, Zeynen B. and Marcia Inhorn, eds. 2011. "Symposium: Cross-Border Reproductive Care – Ethical, Legal, and Socio-Cultural Perspectives." *Reproductive BioMedicine Online* 23 (5): 535–676.

Inhorn, Marcia. 2003. *Local Babies, Global Science: Gender, Religion, and in Vitro Fertilization in Egypt.* New York: Routledge.

———. 2015. *Cosmopolitan Conceptions: IVF Sojourns in Global Dubai.* Durham: Duke University Press.

Inhorn, Marcia and Pasquale Patrizio. 2015. "Infertility around the Globe: New Thinking on Gender, Reproductive Technologies and Global Movements in the 21st Century." *Human Reproduction Update* 21 (4): 411–26.

Ishihara, Osamu and Yasunori Yoshimura. 2011. "Damages at Japanese Assisted Reproductive Technology Clinics by the Great Eastern Japan Earthquake of 2011." *Fertility and Sterility* 95 (8): 2568–70.

Knecht, Michi, Maren Klotz, and Stefan Beck, eds. 2012. *Reproductive Technologies as Global Form: Ethnographies of Knowledge, Practices, and Transnational Encounters.* Frankfurt: Campus Verlag.

Lewis, Ori. 2015. "Israel Evacuates Surrogate-born Babies and Israeli Parents from Nepal." April 27. https://www.reuters.com/article/us-quake-nepal-israel-babies-idUSKBN0NI0RA20150427 (Last accessed September 29, 2018).

Lovett, Natalie. 2017. *Lexie's Village*. Paddington: RZ Publishing.

Luce, Jacqueline. 2010. *Beyond Expectation: Lesbian/Bi/Queer Women and Assisted Conception.* Toronto: University of Toronto Press.

Mackie, Vera. 2009. "Family Law and its Others." In *Japanese Family Law in Comparative Perspective*, edited by Harry Scheiber and Laurent Mayali, 139–63. Berkeley: Robbins Collection.

———. 2013. "Genders and Genetics: The Legal and Medical Regulation of Family Forms in Japan." *Australian Journal of Asian Law* 14 (1): 1–18.

———. 2014a. "Birth Registration and the Right to Have Rights: The Changing Family and the Unchanging Koseki." In *Japan's Household Registration System and Citizenship: Koseki, Identification and Documentation,* edited by David Chapman and Karl J. Krogness, 203–20. London: Routledge.

———. 2014b. "Science, Society and the Sea of Fertility: New Reproductive Technologies in Japanese Popular Culture." *Japan Forum* 26 (4): 441–61.

———. 2018. "Nation, Narration and Family-Making in Australia." Unpublished paper presented at the Workshop on Reproductive Futures in the Asia-Pacific, Monash University, June 2018.

Mackie, Vera and Carolyn S. Stevens. 2009. "Globalisation and Body Politics." *Asian Studies Review* 33 (3): 257–73.

Mamo, Laura. 2007. *Queering Reproduction: Achieving Pregnancy in the Age of Technoscience.* Durham: Duke University Press.

Marks, Nicola J. 2017. "Population, Reproduction and IVF in New Caledonia: Exploring Sociocultural and Caring Dimensions of Sustainable Development." *PORTAL Journal of Multidisciplinary International Studies* 14 (2): 6–26.

Murdoch, Lindsay. 2017. "A Mother's Anguish as Gammy Celebrates Fourth Birthday." *Stuff*, December 24. https://www.stuff.co.nz/life-style/parenting/100156066/a-mothers-anguish-as-gammy-celebrates-fourth-birthday (Last accessed September 29, 2018).

Ottolenghi, Yotam. 2014. "Why I'm Coming Out as a Gay Father." *The Guardian*, August 3. https://www.theguardian.com/lifeandstyle/2013/aug/03/yotam-ottolenghi-gay-fatherhood-parenting (Last accessed September 29, 2018).

Pande, Amrita. 2014. *Wombs in Labor: Transnational Commercial Surrogacy in India.* New York: Columbia University Press.

———. 2016. "Global Reproductive Inequalities, Neo-Eugenics and Commercial Surrogacy in India." *Current Sociology* 64 (2): 244–58.

Rabinow, Paul and Nikolas Rose. 2006. "Biopower Today." *BioSocieties* 1 (2): 195–217.

Rafferty, John P. n.d. "Nepal Earthquake of 2015." *Encyclopædia Britannica.* https://www.britannica.com/topic/Nepal-earthquake-of-2015 (Last accessed July 26, 2018).

Ramzy, Austin. 2018. "Baby in China is Born to Surrogate 4 Years after his Parents' Deaths." *New York Times*, April 12. https://www.nytimes.com/2018/04/12/world/asia/china-baby-dead-parents.html (Last accessed September 29, 2018).

Robertson, John A. 2015. "Surrogacy, Israel, and the Nepal Earthquake." *Harvard Law Bill of Health blog*, June 4. http://blogs.harvard.edu/billofhealth/2015/06/04/surrogacy-israel-and-the-nepal-earthquake/ (Last accessed September 29, 2018).

Rozée, Virginie and Sayeed Unisa, eds. 2016. *Assisted Reproductive Technologies in the Global South and North: Issues, Challenges and the Future.* Oxford: Routledge.

Sarojini, N. and Vrinda Marwah, eds. 2015. *Reconfiguring Reproduction: Feminist Health Perspectives on Assisted Reproductive Technologies.* New Delhi: Sama and Zubaan.

SBS News. 2017. "IVF Tourism: The Chinese Women Travelling to Australia for a Baby." *Insight.* https://www.sbs.com.au/news/ivf-tourism-the-chinese-women-travelling-to-australia-for-a-baby?cx_cid=edm:newspm:2017 (Last accessed July 23, 2018).

Schurr, Carolin. 2016. "From Biopolitics to Bioeconomies: The ART of (re-) producing White Futures in Mexico's Surrogacy Market." *Environment and Planning D: Society and Space* 35 (2): 241–62.

Spar, Debora. 2006. *The Baby Business: How Money, Science, and Politics Drive the Commerce of Conception.* Boston: Harvard Business School Press.
Thompson, Charis. 2005. *Making Parents: The Ontological Choreography of Reproductive Technologies.* Cambridge, MA: MIT Press.
Wade, Katherine. 2017. "The Regulation of Surrogacy: A Children's Rights Perspective." *Child and Family Law Quarterly* 29 (2): 113–31.
Whittaker, Andrea. 2011. "Cross-Border Assisted Reproduction Care in Asia: Implications for Access, Equity and Regulations." *Reproductive Health Matters* 19 (37): 107–16.

Chapter 1

A Tale of Two Halves?

IVF in the UK in the 1970s and 1980s

Sarah Franklin

As Martin Johnson and Kay Elder (2015) describe in their invaluable historical research on in vitro fertilization (IVF) in the United Kingdom, much of what is known about the early period of the development of this technology derives from the writings of Robert Edwards (1925–2013), including his coauthored (with Patrick Steptoe [1913–1988]) book *A Matter of Life* (1980), other books and articles, and now also his notes, laboratory books, and correspondence.[1] In *A Matter of Life*, Edwards and Steptoe trace the journey to the birth of Louise Brown in 1978, the first baby born after conception through IVF. Two other primary historical accounts of Louise Brown's birth in Oldham in 1978 are the memoir by Louise's parents, Lesley and John, written by journalist Sue Freeman, entitled *Our Miracle Called Louise* (1979) and the documentary film produced and directed by Peter Williams in 1978, *To Mrs. Brown a Daughter*. Since the award of a Nobel Prize to Robert Edwards in 2010, followed by his death in 2013, increasing scholarly attention has turned to the historical study of IVF in the United Kingdom. Recently Louise Brown has published an autobiography (2015), and more scholarly articles have been published chronicling the journey from successful fertilization of human ova in Edwards's Cambridge laboratory in 1969 to the delivery of Louise Brown in Oldham nearly a decade later (Elder and Johnson 2015a, 2015b, 2015c; Johnson and Elder 2015a, 2015b, 2015c).

Despite increasing attention to its origins, IVF can be described as a surprisingly understudied technology. IVF is one of the most successful translational technologies of the twentieth century, one that has changed fundamentally the very meaning of "reproduction" (Franklin 2013). Considering its enormous economic, cultural, political, ethical, legal, and social—not to mention medical and scientific—importance, however, surprisingly few research projects have focused on what we might learn from IVF's substantial sociocultural impact. Compared to the number of social and historical studies of the human genome project, for example, IVF's histories and cultures remain largely unmapped. In particular, we know very little about the historical contexts out of which IVF emerged in dozens of countries around the world in the 1980s and 1990s, or even why it emerged the way it did in the United Kingdom. Johnson and Elder's research symposium in *Reproductive Biomedicine and Society Online* (2015) on the Oldham period is one of the only scholarly accounts, other than those of Edwards himself, to provide substantial knowledge about early IVF in the United Kingdom. These publications revealed, among other things, how much more difficult it was both technically and logistically to achieve clinical IVF than previously thought; how many more unsuccessful cycles preceded a successful pregnancy than was previously known; and how substantially early IVF was funded by an anonymous American donor, whose identity Elder and Johnson only recently made known following her death (2015, 63–4). That so many basic details have only recently been published confirms how much work remains to be done in order to place human IVF technology in its historical and social context, and to explain how and why human reproduction was so dramatically transformed in the late twentieth century.

In this chapter, I offer a preliminary sociological map of one aspect of the history of IVF in the United Kingdom which may repay further investigation—especially in the comparative global context this volume seeks to present. The following description contrasts the period of IVF's initial development in Oldham and Cambridge in the 1970s against its rapid growth under Thatcherism in the 1980s, arguing that these two periods represent two substantially different phases in the development of IVF, albeit in the same national context. The aim of this exercise is to argue that we cannot understand either IVF's translational success or its transformative effects, unless we can develop concepts and models that allow us to more fully situate IVF within the social and historical contexts out of which it emerges. There are many different forms of IVF technology, just as IVF itself is a hybrid of several different kinds of technology. These technologies are social too: kinship and gender systems, for example, are two of the most important social technologies through which fertility is both organized and actualized. IVF reproduces more than babies, parents, and families: it reproduces identities and imaginaries, norms and values, goals and aspirations.

As an increasing range of scholarly publications has demonstrated, the infrastructures of nation-states play a crucial role in shaping how IVF and other reproductive technologies, including contraception and abortion, become available and to whom. Religion, research funding and training facilities, public opinion, the media, government, legislatures, and a host of other institutional factors play a role in shaping the "repronational" landscapes within which IVF technology takes a variety of forms worldwide (Franklin and Inhorn 2016). Individuals, such as politicians, clinicians, celebrities, patients, religious leaders, and patient activists, can also change the course of IVF histories in ways that enable us to better understand how IVF technology "works" in social as well as biological, medical, and scientific terms. One important outcome of such an improved understanding is a more robust and multifaceted model of the relationship between technological translation and social context.

IVF in the United Kingdom offers an excellent case study for repronational analysis because it contains an internal contrast that allows us to compare its development in two phases. These two phases are divided by the radical socio-political transformation of the United Kingdom that coincided almost exactly with the birth of Louise Brown, namely the birth of "Thatcherism" and the "enterprise culture." During the 1970s, research on IVF in Oldham took place under the well-established British ethos of national social welfare, driven by an aspirational optimism and a collective commitment to human betterment that was supported by a state which promoted medical and technological progress. The ideals of the Oldham team reflected the progressive spirit of the postwar British welfare state, and its liberal humanitarian commitment to health and welfare, epitomized by the 1942 Beveridge Report's ambitious proposal of a universal guarantee of support "from cradle to grave." The centerpiece of this legislation, the 1946 National Health Service Act, established for the first time the legal principle of universal health entitlement. Both the architects of Beveridge's reforms, and the expanded welfare support services of the post–Second World War period, encouraged and rewarded a spirit of altruistic voluntarism. This was demonstrated by the "army" of "ovum pioneers" in Oldham, which included not only the large numbers of altruistically motivated women patients but also the large staff of nurses and technicians who supported them—often for no pay. Robert Edwards, a lifelong socialist, and Jean Purdy (1945–1985), a dedicated former nurse, worked alongside Patrick Steptoe—a highly committed National Health Service (NHS) consultant obstetrician—and his large team of support staff in the Oldham General Infirmary. A strong sense of teamwork and a sustained collective ambition to succeed against the odds were essential during the long, inadequately funded, understaffed, poorly equipped, and logistically daunting period of repeated IVF failure for nearly a decade prior to Louise Brown's birth in 1978.

The Conservative prime minister Margaret Thatcher (1925–2013) was elected in 1979, the year following Louise Brown's birth in Lancashire in July 1978, and a very different role for IVF soon emerged in the United Kingdom. Somewhat ironically, given its origins under the National Health Service, IVF was transformed into a bellwether of health privatization. From its birth as a technique intended to improve the options for infertile couples, and to further medical science, IVF in Britain soon acquired a very different role as a lucrative private health service blazing a new trail in the "enterprise culture" of Thatcher's Britain in the 1980s (Franklin 1997). Redefined as consumer-citizens under Thatcher's newly individualized concept of the social contract linking "stakeholders" to the British government, the socialist ideals of universal health and welfare which dominated the 1970s were supplanted by a new conservatism, characterized by an emergent neoliberal demonization of the so-called nanny state and its attendant burdens on the British taxpayer. I chart this process below to illustrate how IVF was incorporated into national political strategies of governance. In the United Kingdom, as elsewhere, IVF can serve this function particularly well because it continues to be a powerful symbolic technology for governments as well as other constituencies. In this way, I further develop the concept of "repronationalism" while situating IVF in the United Kingdom within a comparative global frame (Franklin and Inhorn 2016).

EARLY IVF

Oldham is both an out-of-the-way and historically significant town in the heavily industrialized Northwest region of England. It was here in Lancashire that the Industrial Revolution began in the mid-eighteenth century, where the canals and railways enabled an unprecedented density of commodity production and distribution, and great commercial wealth was accumulated off the backs of a proletarian populace known equally for their staunch regional pride and their capacity to endure extreme working conditions.[2] Many of the patients at the Oldham General Infirmary came from large working-class families whose mill-working ancestors would have witnessed high levels of childhood and maternal mortality, widespread malnutrition, and long hours of factory labor, resulting in short life expectancies. The Northwest is also a region renowned for social and technological innovation—and for progressive social movements, high levels of civic enterprise, and free trade halls. The unshowy and anti-establishment Northern ethos derived from such legacies combines the proverbial British stiff upper lip with a pragmatic approach to overcoming obstacles, often through a combination of ingenuity and persistence. This region is as strongly characterized by the productive linkages between agriculture and industry that have shaped its utilitarian landscapes as by its rejection of the courtly codes of the aristocracy, which reflect an older order of wealth generation and inherited privilege.

During the post–Second World War period, maternal and childhood morbidity diminished significantly in the United Kingdom from the high rates seen as late as the 1950s. Average family size had reduced accordingly.

From 1900 to 1935, the average maternal mortality rate in England was 400 per 100,000 births. By 1980, this rate had declined to fewer than 9 deaths per 100,000 births (Loudon 1992). The postwar introduction of the NHS shifted much of the health and social care work formerly provided by charitable organizations such as the Mothers' Union into the formal apparatus of the state. Major medical scientific contributions such as the introduction of antibiotics, in combination with greatly improved nutrition and housing, produced very different conditions from those prevailing for much of the first half of the twentieth century in towns like Oldham. The nationalization of healthcare and the implementation of science-based means of improving health and welfare invited further forms of modernization—to which Steptoe responded with a catalog of new inventions aimed at reducing age-old problems such as the termination of unwanted pregnancy (Pickstone 1985, 253).

When he arrived in Oldham in 1951, after a short stint in the Navy, Patrick Steptoe initially encountered a considerable backlog of cases, including classic sequellae of under-diagnosis such as large ovarian tumors and severe uterine prolapses among his catchment population of 300,000. "This initially took up all his time, as he worked seven days per week to catch up until the situation was brought under far better control," said Robert Edwards in his biographical memoir of Steptoe (Edwards 1996, 437). Although Lancashire had a strong tradition of voluntary hospital service prior to the enactment of the National Health Act in 1948, "textile towns" like Oldham had been hit hard by economic depression between the wars, and only one new large hospital was built in the Lancashire region between the outbreak of the First World War and the establishment of the National Health Service (NHS). "For the rest, the history of voluntary hospitals between the wars was mostly a succession of extensions on increasingly crowded sites . . . usually paid for by special appeals, bazaars, fund-raising concerts, etc." (Pickstone 1985, 253). This lack of increase in hospital facilities between the wars was in spite of a significant expansion in their workload, including an increase from 2,000 in-patients per annum in 1918 to 7,000 in 1938. The number of outpatients rose from 5,600 to 36,500, and surgical operations increased tenfold (Pickstone 1985, 254–55).

As Martin Johnson and Kay Elder have documented (and as Edwards himself discusses in many of his published works), successful IVF relied on many patients volunteering to undergo laparoscopic egg extraction with no prospect of embryo transfer (97 patients underwent 159 laparoscopic surgeries that were of no potential benefit to the patient). According to interview data from nurses and patients who were in Oldham in the 1970s, as well as Edwards' own accounts, it appears the consent procedures for such operations—although not as rigorous as they would be today—made it clear that there was no prospect of individual success, and that participation was intended for the greater good of improving the technique. A considerable degree of selflessness and faith in medical progress, as well as physical stamina and high tolerance of personal risk, was thus required of the large, entirely female, volunteer "army" of "ovum pioneers" whose willingness to undergo experimental treatment with little or no chance of benefiting from it themselves paved the way to successful IVF (Elder and Johnson 2015a, 2015b, 2015c; Johnson and Elder 2015d, 2015e, 2015f).

Steptoe's early work with laparoscopy reflected the poor state of reproductive care he initially encountered in Oldham, and his new surgical method appears in no small part to have been motivated by a desire to alleviate the suffering of patients who had to endure lengthy and costly hospital stays to undergo either basic abdominal investigations or simple procedures such as tubal ligation.[3] In a letter in 1966 to the *British Medical Journal* (Steptoe 1966, 234) Steptoe makes a compelling case for the superiority of laparoscopic diathermy to other forms of contraception and sterilization. While urging appropriate care in the use of such irreversible measures, and acknowledging the potential for their misuse, Steptoe persuasively argues for the advantages this method offers over any other in achieving effective permanent sterility in those cases where it is genuinely sought. Contraception, he argues, may well be effective for the spacing of children, but not as a permanent means of preventing them, for example, when a desired family size has been reached. In contrast to the many disadvantages of the contraceptive pill and the IUD, and the inadequacies of many existing means of sterilization (the Madlener operation, the Pomroy method), laparoscopic surgery delivers superior results with less preparation, shorter anesthesia, lower cost, faster recovery, and fewer complications, he stated.[4]

In this way, Steptoe, like Edwards, belonged to a distinctively modern, post–Second World War, Euro-American, mid-twentieth-century ethos of progressive scientific improvement in aid of improved human health, facilitated by new technologies, modern health services, and government support. This goal was energetically sought through (often publicly funded) research programs which combined basic science with clinical experimentation to develop frontier applications of technologies that today would be described as "translational." Although inevitably beset by some degree of disagreement as to the best way forward, this broad ethos was generally understood to be virtuous, beneficent, and consensual. It is a modern progressive ethos epitomized by the "endless frontier" analogy in the 1945 Franklin Delano Roosevelt and Vannever Bush manifesto commissioning the swords-into-ploughshares transfer of military spending into healthcare (Bush 1945). This promise was symbolically embodied in the United States by the establishment of the National Science Foundation (NSF). The same promise of scientifically improved health, as a response to the tragic loss of life in the Second World

War, is enshrined in the gift, sacrifice, and reparation analogies accompanying the formation of the British NHS in 1948. Control of reproduction was central to both of these postwar national health improvement strategies, and indeed comprised a major focus of political, philanthropic, economic, medical, and scientific endeavor worldwide during the 1960s and 1970s (Clarke 1998).[5]

As the historian Alison Bashford argues, war, migration, and concerns about the environment were already linked to the scientific effort to improve health—through the many Malthusian models deployed by scientists, politicians, and social reformers throughout the twentieth century (Bashford 2016). These concerns reached their apex in the form of increasingly global concerns about the population "bomb" that peaked in the 1970s—directly prior to IVF's first successes "in man". As the goal of more scientifically controlled reproduction became ever more central to international politics from 1945 onward, it became the focus of increasing scientific attention. It was by this means that large-scale political, economic, and national security concerns about population growth were translated into the first popular reproductive technologies in countries such as the United Kingdom, where the oral contraceptive pill was introduced in 1971 (and legalized in 1974, see Pfeffer 1993). So too did the concept of reproductive rights become linked to both human rights and women's rights in this period of substantial economic growth accompanied by rapid social liberalization.

In Britain, as in the United States, the late 1960s was a period dominated by progressive social change—much of it driven by activist social movements. The (socialist) Labour Party came into power with a large majority following the 1966 General Election, inaugurating a lengthy period of progressive reform in British politics. Labour leader Harold Wilson was elected prime minister in 1964, after thirteen years of Conservative government, and remained in office until 1970, returning to lead again in 1974. In the same year, he was succeeded by James Callaghan, who extended the Labour government's leadership until Margaret Thatcher's election in 1979.[6] Feminism became much more prominent during this period, as did the struggle for free and legal abortion, which emerged as a defining issue for the women's liberation movement (WLM) in many advanced industrial countries, including Britain. Indeed, the campaign to reform abortion law, culminating in the 1967 Abortion Act, continues to be seen as a watershed in British politics, epitomizing to many commentators the successful reforms of the 1960s which emerged out of progressive social movements for equal rights.

Before the 1967 Act, an average of fifty women a year would die from "back street" abortions in the United Kingdom, while countless others suffered severe health consequences. Even those who could pay for the comparatively safe option of arranging for a termination with a highly skilled and respected consultant such as Patrick Steptoe did so under a thick layer of social stigma that permeated the medical profession itself. The Abortion Act significantly transformed both the accessibility of abortion and social attitudes toward unwanted pregnancy. It radically reconstituted national reproductivity in legislative, moral, demographic, and personal terms. In 1969, 50,000 abortions were performed in the United Kingdom. Just over a decade later, in 1983, more than twice as many were performed annually (127,000) (Mulkay 1997, 8).

The decriminalization of abortion dramatically altered childbearing patterns at both an aggregate and an individual level. As new options emerged, others were foreclosed with immediate and substantial consequences for the social organization of parenthood. British sociologist Michael Mulkay describes this change as preconditional to the later surge in demand for IVF services in the 1980s. He argues that "during the 1970s, the legislative success of the pro-abortion lobby . . . in conjunction with underlying demographic trends, helped to increase the potential demand for a technological solution to the problem of childlessness within marriage" (1997, 9). As the number of abortions more than doubled, the number of unwanted pregnancies taken to term more than halved, and the number of babies available for adoption lessened accordingly, thus reducing the supply of children available for adoption at precisely the time more childless couples were seeking to adopt them. In 1966 approximately 25,000 adoptions took place per annum, and within a decade this number halved to 13,000. Within two years of the adoption of the 1967 Abortion Act, one-third of voluntary adoption agencies in Britain had closed (Mulkay 1997, 9).

The rapidly changing landscape of reproductive behavior during the 1970s was not only driven by legislative, demographic, and technological factors; it was also shaped by a moral and cultural revolt, reflecting and expressing the declining influence of so-called Victorian moral values, as well as increasing support for women's rights. This change was the result of affective as well as political shifts, such as increasing social intolerance of the moral shame and stigma associated with "illegitimate" pregnancy. Within less than a decade, the 1967 Abortion Act had all but eliminated the conventional and institutionalized reproductive transaction whereby unmarried women carried their offspring to term before giving them up to "legitimate" and "deserving" childless married couples for adoption.

In mid-Victorian England, one woman in three was unmarried, and the disproportionate number of women to men was exacerbated by the two World Wars. Only in the 1960s was the gender balance reestablished. This meant that there was a significant increase in the number of women able to marry and to legitimately give birth to children in wedlock, and "one major consequence of this dramatic increase in the proportion of married women in British society,"

Mulkay notes, "was *a significant social relocation* of involuntary infertility from the unmarried to the married population" (1997, 10, emphasis added). Both this change in the way reproduction was socially organized and the language Mulkay uses to describe it—as a "relocation" of infertility from one population to another—point to the complex task of situating the emergence of IVF in the United Kingdom in the 1970s in relation to wider patterns of social and demographic change. Mulkay's point is that the "involuntary infertility" socially imposed upon women unable to marry before the 1970s was "relocated" afterward to infertile married couples, who could no longer turn to the semi-institutionalized supply chain of infants given up by unwed mothers for adoption. In this way, the social organization of British reproduction changed—including the patterns of infertility awareness and provision driven by new distributions of unwanted childlessness, changing attitudes toward parenthood, and new medical options to alleviate infertility. The socially mandated childlessness of unmarried women—whether they bore children or not—in response to the perceived moral stigma of illegitimacy in the 1950s and 1960s was succeeded by a completely different definition of a baby problem for a new group of people in the 1970s. Fertility and infertility were thus reconstituted: for married couples unable to conceive a child of their own, infertility became a problem open to a technological solution.

Mulkay speculates that the significant shifts in the constitution and distribution of postwar fertility patterns were themselves a significant force in the "birth" of IVF. He argues that

> Edwards and his partners were aware from their work in the hospital that the problem of infertility was being made worse by the fall in the adoption rate. They also sensed that, once people came to believe that a science based remedy for infertility was available the demand for their services would grow rapidly. Because they were dealing with married couples, Edwards and his colleagues were confident about their own moral position. (1997, 10)

Consequently, Mulkay concludes, Louise Brown's birth was not only a technological tipping point but also a condensed moment of social and cultural conversion: "the birth of Louise Brown . . . transformed the latent demand for a technological solution to the problem of childlessness into an active demand for the new techniques of assisted reproduction" (1997, 11).

In summarizing the structural and institutional changes during the period directly preceding IVF's initial clinical success in Oldham, specific intersecting forces can usefully be identified. These factors help to explain the emergence of both a demand for IVF and a growing (if highly contested) perception of its moral legitimacy and social value in the United Kingdom. At the national level, a commitment to scientifically based solutions to health and welfare became increasingly prominent in the postwar period. Locally, the NHS took on an increasing responsibility for healthcare, including the new legal options of both abortion and contraception. The moral economy of the nation also shifted dramatically in favor of more tolerant and progressive attitudes toward sexuality and marriage, manifest in more liberal attitudes toward divorce, homosexuality, and single motherhood. The women's movement and other struggles for greater civil rights gained momentum during a period which was also characterized by greater economic prosperity and significant improvements in health and life expectancy. These changes were in many ways encapsulated by the passage of the 1967 Abortion Act, which resulted in yet further social, political, moral, and demographic changes in the 1970s.

As a result of these shifts, Britain's reproductive patterns were significantly reconstituted. Its repronational economy no longer contained a semi-institutionalized supply chain of children given up by unwed mothers for adoption by married couples facing unwanted childlessness. Increasing access to contraception and abortion accompanied by higher rates of marriage and better medical care produced a new demographic effect. More married couples faced fertility problems in a context of fewer children to adopt. In an era which was already increasingly concerned with "disciplining" reproduction (Clarke 1997), the conversion of technologies aimed at the reduction of fertility into the reduction of infertility was fast becoming a reproductive logic with far-reaching consequences. The birth of Louise Brown effected a further conversion—of hope for a technological solution to infertility into a mass consumer market for IVF. As a consequence, Britain's repronational history took yet another complicated turn.

THE "ENTERPRISING UP" OF REPRODUCTION

When Margaret Thatcher came to power in 1979, her election as prime minister ended a lengthy period of Labour dominance of British politics and introduced a new form of Conservative government—one that the Marxist cultural theorist Stuart Hall described as "authoritarian populism" (1988). Key to the political ideology that came to be known as "Thatcherism" was a combination of antagonism toward the so-called dependency culture fostered by the British welfare state with the promotion of a new ethos of enterprising individualism aimed at reducing taxpayer spending on social services. The cornerstones of Thatcherite ideology rested on a commitment to dismantling state-sponsored care schemes, privatization of the national industries and housing stock, and promotion of competitive private enterprise as a moral and national good. This enterprising model of citizenship and the national economy was rooted in a prescriptive model of the family as the primary site of consumer identity. Thatcher argued that the nuclear family should be the fundamental unit of society—and indeed *should replace* the very concept of "society" as the frame of reference within which individuals understood their activities, aspirations, and livelihoods.[7] Thatcher's motto was that there was "no such thing as society, there are only individuals and their families" (Keay 1987). Her aim was to produce a "share-owning democracy" by encouraging a "nation of home-owners" and thus to redefine British citizenship in terms of the market principles of production and consumption. A shopkeeper's daughter herself, she sought to shift the national self-image away from the "nanny" model of a collective citizenship living within a caring state, toward a "stakeholder" nation of more self-reliant individuals who adopted market principles as moral common sense. Championing greater individual prosperity in a culture of increased market freedom, Thatcher's ultimate analogy for 1980s Britain was the modern supermarket—a palace of consumer choice, where people shopped for themselves as well as their families (Franklin, Lury, and Stacey 1991).

Thatcher's vision of a new sense of national belonging forged among competitive individuals striving on behalf of their families guided her radical dismantling of the welfare state infrastructure. Between 1979 and 1990, her government privatized much of the national housing stock. Millions of council house residents purchased their homes at knockdown prices and saw their values more than triple in worth. Accompanying this revolutionary change in the economic fortunes of the largely working-class population of council house owners who had formerly been tenants was a huge rise in mortgage debt. This increased from £45 to £275 billion over the first ten years of Thatcher's leadership. By selling off British Petroleum, British Aerospace, British Telecom, and British Gas during this same period,[8] Thatcher effectively rewrote the social contract between citizens and the British state, transforming it into a financial relationship between individuals, property, and the market. The new form of belonging was not based on the reciprocal principles of all for one and one for all. It was based on shareholding: Thatcher's new description of a citizen was as a "share-holding individual."

Following Thatcher's violent suppression of the national miners' strike during 1984–1985, she accelerated her program of fiscal conservatism by further deregulating the economy, cutting social services, and promoting free trade. Whereas her policies of selling off the national industries and housing stock had won her many new supporters (including many former Labour voters), she was on much more dangerous ground in her efforts to reform the NHS. Still the largest employer in the European Union today, and one of the most advanced and efficient health services in the world, the NHS is also a source of significant national pride and the subject of a unique affection among the British population. The National Health Service is not only an institution but also a symbol of the British values of decency, fairness, and justice. It also symbolizes generosity. In the form of the NHS, the United Kingdom still demonstrates its long-standing commitment to the Labour (socialist) principles that shaped the immediate aftermath of the two World Wars. The NHS was explicitly conceived as a gift to the population in the wake of their enormous sacrifices, and thus as a form of domestic reparation. It symbolizes a commitment to caring for the less well-off, for those in need, and indeed for all citizens regardless of their circumstances.

Since she could not entirely privatize the NHS, Thatcher tried to marketize it piecemeal from within—offering consultants new contracts, for example, which gave them greater freedom to see patients privately for a fee. Thatcher also encouraged the growth of private healthcare schemes by providing attractive tax breaks. By 1988 this sector had doubled in size, attracting more than 2 million new subscribers (Pearson 1992, 221). Ultimately the rise of the so-called two-tier health system—in which those who could afford to pay received better access to healthcare—generated increasingly bitter dissent and came to symbolize the iniquitous legacy of Thatcher's "enterprise culture." This risky strategy of partial NHS privatization ultimately played a significant role in the Conservative Party's nefarious dethroning of their very own "Iron Lady."

The "enterprising up" of reproduction described by Marilyn Strathern in both *After Nature* (1992a) and *Reproducing the Future* (1992b) refers to the neat fit between the emergence of a new market in IVF services and the changes to the organization of health and welfare in the United Kingdom in the 1980s under Thatcherism. As Naomi Pfeffer notes in her account of this period, gynecologists were among the most enterprising medical professionals to take advantage of both the increasing ease of marketing private healthcare and the lucrative financial rewards of serving a newly constituted clientele of would-be parents. In Pfeffer's words, IVF had "transformed . . . the balance sheet of gynaecology beyond all recognition" (1993, 166) by the mid-1980s. This period saw an explosion in IVF provision. By 1986, twenty-three clinics offered IVF in the United Kingdom (VLA 1986) and within five years this number had risen to sixty-four (Pfeffer 1993, 166). Although the majority of these clinics were private, many of them piggybacked on NHS hospitals, where access to surgical theaters and hospital beds avoided the need for costly investments in infrastructure, and services from nursing staff and laboratory facilities could be commissioned at significantly discounted (subsidized) cost. These "semi-private" arrangements, despite having been enabled by legislation aimed at making the NHS more efficient, in fact encouraged the service to be exploited for private financial gain. By 1991, only three UK IVF clinics existed in the public sector. The remaining sixty-one were either wholly private or semiprivate services offered for profit.

In contrast to the 1950s, when Steptoe arrived in Oldham to establish an NHS practice in obstetrics and gynecology, the entire landscape of reproductive options had changed dramatically when Steptoe and Edwards opened their Bourn Hall clinic near Cambridge in the 1980s. Whereas the 1970s NHS had been oriented toward an inclusive ethos of care and repair, the Thatcherite NHS of the 1980s was modeled on a social contract drawn from the free market—where competition was prized as a moral and financial good. Moreover, the emergence of IVF in the United Kingdom was not merely a consequence of these trends but also helped to shape and drive major shifts in the ways in/fertility, technology, governance, and welfare were defined as the twentieth century came to a close.

CONCLUSION

Although this chapter has only begun to sketch a contrast between two divergent phases in the development of IVF in the United Kingdom, and although the contrast may be overdrawn in places, three larger arguments can nonetheless be gleaned from this case study. These have relevance not only to the overarching purposes of this volume but also to the study of technology, modernity, and social change more broadly. The first of these is that IVF's divergent global histories are not merely symptomatic of the variations in national context—such as different systems of law, morality, politics, or religion—but can be read as national histories in their own right as well. This is the meaning of the term "repronationalism," which refers not to the passive way in which IVF is shaped by local circumstances, but to the active ways in which the governance of IVF is used to shape national politics, morality, foreign policy, and the economy. In other words, official national policies about IVF and other reproductive technologies concern not only fertility and demography, or medical ethics, but also the basic principles structuring health and welfare systems, and even the core definition of the social contract linking citizens to the state. From this perspective, IVF provides a unique and arguably under-recognized vantage point from which to appreciate that, as Laura Briggs argues, "all politics are reproductive politics" (2017, 14). The second, and related, argument is that placing "the lens of IVF" at the center of social analysis helps us to interpret phenomena such as Thatcherism, and its emphasis on the promotion of private fertility care within the "enterprise culture" ethos of individual consumers purchasing "free market" goods on behalf of themselves and their families—independently of a "nanny" welfare state, and instead funded by the dividends they receive as shareholders in formerly nationalized industries such as coal, gas, oil, electricity, and rail and air travel. Indeed, it would be hard to find a better condensation of these disparate components of Thatcher's enterprise culture than the private and highly profitable

IVF sector. The final argument is that fertility and infertility are not simply fluctuating biological states which occur more or less independently of social factors but instead are socially shaped—or "constituted." As is especially clear in retrospect, changing fertilities and infertilities are products of history. The shifts in morality and politics which reconfigured marriage and parenting patterns in 1950s Britain helped to establish "fertile ground" for the birth of IVF; and the emergence of the vast and largely private fertility industry we see growing so rapidly in the early twenty-first century is in turn a product of a political climate that favored "free market" fertility care. Understanding the patterns through which fertilities and infertilities are constituted—morally, politically, technologically, and economically—is crucial to the process of appreciating how the constitution of fertilities and infertilities shapes morality, politics, translational science, and the economy. These are lessons it will be increasingly important to understand in the coming decades during which reproductive politics will increasingly move to center stage worldwide.

NOTES

1. The research for this chapter was funded by a combination of grants from the Wellcome Trust, the Economic and Social Research Council (ESRC), the British Academy, Christ's College, and the University of Cambridge (Vice-Chancellor's Fund).

2. Marx and Engels based much of their account of the Industrial Revolution in Manchester, a few miles from Oldham.

3. Laparoscopy involves making a small incision in the abdomen and is less invasive than other procedures in use at the time.

4. In other articles from this period, Steptoe advocates the use of laparoscopy for numerous other purposes, including combined termination and sterilization (Steptoe and Imran 1969, 751–52), and in general he was actively and experimentally engaged in the effort to deliver better and more scientifically informed approaches to both reduce maternal morbidity and address the pressing issue of population control—considered in the 1960s and the 1970s to be of paramount importance to the improvement of human futures.

5. "The new sciences of embryology" also feature prominently in feminist works of this period, most notably that of Shulamith Firestone (1970), who referred to it variously as "the new population biology," "modern embryology" and "control of human fertility."

6. Thatcher remained prime minister for ten years until John Major succeeded her, and he led the Conservatives until the Labour Party was returned to power in 1991 under the leadership of Tony Blair.

7. Thatcher's family model did not include a reversion to the so-called Victorian values of a previous era, or to its neo-patriarchalism. Although the election of a Tory government encouraged many right-wing activists and groups to resume an attack on

the liberal reforms of the 1960s and 1970s, and Thatcher did little to oppose them, she and her governments largely kept their distance from the key issues of abortion, censorship, contraception, homosexuality, and civil rights which had been the subjects of progressive reform under Labour.

8. Thatcher also auctioned off Rolls Royce, Cable and Wireless (the nation's telegraph and telecommunications companies), the water companies, the airports, and the shipping ports.

WORKS CITED

Bashford, Alison. 2016. *Global Population: History, Geopolitics, and Life on Earth.* New York: Columbia University Press.

Briggs, Laura. 2017. *How All Politics Became Reproductive Politics: From Welfare Reform to Foreclosure to Trump.* Berkeley: University of California Press.

Brown, Lesley and John Brown, with Sue Freeman. 1979. *Our Miracle Called Louise.* New York: Paddington Press.

Brown, Louise and Martin Powell. 2015. *Louise Brown: My Life as the World's First Test-Tube Baby.* United Kingdom: Bristol Books.

Bush, Vannevar. 1945. *Science the Endless Frontier: A Report to the President by Vannevar Bush, Director of the Office of Scientific Research and Development.* Washington, DC: United States Government Printing Office.

Edwards, Robert. 1989. *Life Before Birth: Reflections on the Embryo Debate.* London: Angus and Robertson.

Edwards, Robert G. and Patrick C. Steptoe. 1980. *A Matter of Life: The Story of a Medical Breakthrough.* London: Angus and Robertson.

Elder, Kay and Martin H. Johnson. 2015a. "The Oldham Notebooks: An Analysis of the Development of IVF 1969–1978. I. Introduction, Materials and Methods." *Reproductive Biomedicine & Society Online* 1 (1): 3–8.

———. 2015b. "The Oldham Notebooks: An Analysis of the Development of IVF 1969–1978. II. The Treatment Cycles and Their Outcomes." *Reproductive Biomedicine & Society* 1 (1): 9–18.

———. 2015c. "The Oldham Notebooks: An Analysis of the Development of IVF 1969–1978. III. Variations in Procedures." *Reproductive Biomedicine & Society Online* 1 (1): 19–33.

Firestone, Shulamith. 1970. *The Dialectic of Sex: The Case for Feminist Revolution.* New York: William Morris and Company.

Franklin, Sarah. 1997. *Embodied Progress: A Cultural Analysis of Assisted Conception.* London: Routledge.

———. 2013. *Biological Relatives: IVF, Stem Cells, and the Future of Kinship. North Carolina.* Duke University Press.

Franklin, Sarah and Marcia Inhorn, eds. 2016. "Symposium: IVF - Global Histories." *Reproductive Biomedicine & Society Online* 2: 1–136.

Franklin, Sarah, Celia Lury, and Jackie Stacey. 2000. *Global Nature, Global Culture.* London: Sage.

Hall, Stuart. 1988. "The Toad in the Garden: Thatcherism among the Theorists." In *Marxism and the Interpretation of Culture*, edited by Cary Nelson and Lawrence Grossberg, 35–74. Basingstoke: Macmillan.

Johnson, Martin. 2011. "Robert Edwards: The Path to IVF." *Reproductive Biomedicine Online* 23 (2): 245–62.

Johnson, Martin H. and Kay Elder. 2015a. "The Oldham Notebooks: An Analysis of the Development of IVF 1969–1978 V. The Role of Jean Purdy Reassessed." *Reproductive Biomedicine & Society* 1 (1): 46–57.

———. 2015b. "The Oldham Notebooks: An Analysis of the Development of IVF 1969–1978. IV. Ethical Aspects." *Reproductive Biomedicine & Society* 1 (1): 34–45.

———. 2015c. "The Oldham Notebooks: An Analysis of the Development of IVF 1969–1978. VI. Sources of Support and Patterns of Expenditure." *Reproductive Biomedicine & Society* 1 (1): 58–70.

Johnson, Martin H., Sarah B. Franklin, M. Cottingham, and N. Hopwood. 2010. "Why the Medical Research Council Refused Robert Edwards and Patrick Steptoe Support for Research on Human Conception in 1971." *Human Reproduction* 25: 2157–74.

Keay, Douglas. 1987. "Interview for *Women's Own*: "No Such Thing as Society." Interview with Margaret Thatcher. *Women's Own*, September 23, 1987. https://www.margaretthatcher,org/document/106689 (Last accessed January 7, 2018).

Loudon, Irvine. 1992. "The Transformation of Maternal Mortality." *British Medical Journal* 305: 1557–60.

Mulkay, Michael. 1997. *The Embryo Research Debate: Science and the Politics of Reproduction*. Cambridge, England: Cambridge University Press.

Pfeffer, Naomi. 1993. *The Stork and the Syringe: A Political History of Reproductive Medicine*. Cambridge: Polity Press.

Pickstone John. 1985. *Medicine and Industrial Society: A History of Hospital Development in Manchester and its Region, 1752–1946*. Manchester: Manchester University Press.

Steptoe, Patrick. 1966. "The Fifth Freedom." *British Medical Journal* 1 (5481): 234.

Steptoe, Patrick and M. Imran. 1969. "Combined Procedure of Aspiration Termination and Laparoscopic Sterilization." *British Medical Journal* 27 (September): 751–52.

Strathern, Marilyn. 1992a. *After Nature: English Kinship in the Late Twentieth Century*. Cambridge: Cambridge University Press.

______. 1992b. *Reproducing the Future: Essays on Anthropology, Kinship and the New Reproductive Technologies*. Manchester: Manchester University Press.

To Mrs. Brown a Daughter. 1978. Directed by Peter Williams. United Kingdom: Thames Television.

Chapter 2

Situating India in the Global Reproductive Industry

Vasudha Mohanka

In this chapter, I trace the development of the reproductive services industry in India and situate it in the context of the global reproductive industry. All nation-states manage their populations in various ways, either through pronatalist policies which encourage reproduction, policies on population limitation, or policies which encourage or discourage reproduction in particular groups. Foucault's concepts of biopolitics and biopower have been employed by several scholars to analyze governments' control over populations through various mechanisms (Foucault 1978; Nadimpally, Marwah, and Shenoi 2011; Mackie 2014a). The concept of "repronationalism," whereby countries use reproductive policies to shape and express national identity, is also relevant (Franklin 2016; Franklin in this volume). Analytical concepts such as "repronational histories" and "repronational choreographies" are useful to understand patterns of "specific national events" in the context of assisted reproduction (Franklin and Inhorn 2016). Such concepts can be applied to the nature of state interventions in India, the regulation of reproductive services, and more recent attempts to shape national identity through the creation of a particular type of heteronormative family using reproductive technologies like IVF and, in some circumstances, surrogacy arrangements. Reproduction now takes place in a global frame, with intending parents crossing national borders to access gametes and reproductive services. This means that biopolitical interventions by particular governments also have repercussions across national borders, as we shall see below.

From the mid-twentieth century, India has been subject to policies which encourage population limitation, supported by such organizations as the World Health Organization and the International Planned Parenthood Federation (IPPF). Population control schemes looked at "human beings not as individuals but as populations that could be shaped through the combined force of faith and science" (Connelly 2008, xii). From the latter half of the twentieth century, however, increased attention has been paid to facilitating reproduction for some people through assisted reproduction.

In the decades since the first IVF birth in India in 1978, a burgeoning domestic reproductive health services industry has developed. While infertility management in India started primarily in the public sector, it gradually moved to the private sector, albeit with state facilitation (Bharadwaj 2016a, 2002; Sengupta 2010). India has also become a destination country for medical travel including, until the recent enactment of the Surrogacy Regulation Bill (Government of India 2018), travel for reproductive services.

There are several reasons for the growth in reproductive services in the late twentieth and early twenty-first centuries, especially of transnational medical travel to India. The country has state-of-the-art facilities and infrastructure, especially in private fertility and IVF clinics, English-speaking medical professionals trained in prestigious medical schools in India and abroad, cost-effectiveness, attractive tourist destinations, the growth of corporate hospitals and chains, support for medical travel in public policy, attractive deals and offers, and until recently a relative absence of regulation. There is a large population of Indians overseas who have combined medical treatment with a family visit (Sengupta 2008; Nadimpally, Marwah, and Shenoi 2011; Pande 2011). The Indian government provides incentives to clinics by providing low interest rates to establish hospitals and subsidies for buying drugs, importing equipment, and purchasing land (Nadimpally, Marwah, and Shenoi 2011).

In this chapter, I trace the chronological history of human IVF in India and the development of the domestic reproductive health industry, particularly private clinics. Parallel socioeconomic developments led to India becoming a destination for medical and reproductive travel. Controversies concerning transnational surrogacy arrangements then led to calls for further regulation. Finally, I outline recent government policies on regulating reproductive technologies, especially transnational commercial gestational surrogacy.

THE BEGINNINGS

IVF developed through a series of scientific developments from the late nineteenth century. Once the mechanisms of fertilization were understood, they gradually became open to manipulation by medical practitioners. Powerful microscopes allowed scientists to actually observe the fertilization process. Artificial insemination by donor was one step in the separation of fertilization, implantation, and gestation (Brinsden 2011, 3; Bavister 2002; Clarke 2006). Colin Austin (1914–2004) and M. C. Chang (1908–1991) were among the first to discover the need for the spermatozoa to undergo capacitation.[1] Chang's study in 1959 showed that despite a low proportion of fertilized ova, they had "a repeatable procedure for fertilizing mammalian ova *in vitro* and that such ova [were] truly fertilized and able to develop into normal young" (Chang 1959, 467). In other studies live births were achieved after hamster oocytes were fertilized using "spermatozoa capacitated in vitro" (Yanagimachi and Chang 1964, 1963; Bavister 2002). These studies were crucial to the development of human IVF (Bavister 2002).

A series of developments in the United Kingdom, Australia, and other countries led to the development of IVF. Researchers in these countries at times competed and at other times collaborated with each other. Robert Edwards's (1925–2013) team made one of the earliest observations of the fertilization of human oocytes. Edwards's need for collaboration to obtain oocytes brought him in contact with gynecologist Patrick Steptoe (1913–1988) in the year 1968 (Johnson 2011, 254). Steptoe, who developed the technique of laparoscopy,[2] later produced various landmark scientific papers with Edwards.

Following successful IVF and embryo culture studies in animals, presented and discussed at the Australian Society for Reproductive Biology Conference in 1970, Neil Moore suggested to Carl Wood (1929–2011) that they could use a similar approach for the treatment of infertility in humans. After observing Moore and his then PhD student Alan Trounson, Carl Wood (1929–2011) established a research team in Melbourne which included Ian Johnston from the Royal Women's Hospital, John Leeton and James Talbot from the Queen Victoria Medical Centre, and Alex Lopata from Monash University (Cohen et al. 2005).

For nearly a decade between 1968 and 1978, Edwards and Steptoe made numerous attempts to transfer embryos created through IVF, resulting in one ectopic pregnancy and 102 failed embryo transfers. Following this, Lesley Brown became pregnant after her first embryo transfer achieved "in a 'natural' IVF cycle, with no stimulation." Following a difficult pregnancy, Lesley gave birth to a healthy Louise Brown by caesarean section on July 25, 1978 (Brinsden 2011, 4). The Edwards-Steptoe team in the United Kingdom had a "bumpy road," though, in relation to the development of in vitro fertilization due to lack of funding and other problems (Gallagher 2013; Murthy 2010; Franklin in this volume). Murthy highlights the opposition to their research from various groups such as the Roman Catholic Church and scientists who were skeptical of the technology because they believed that the children might be born with abnormalities. Ethical considerations were another significant reason for the road being "bumpy" for Edwards and Steptoe (Murthy 2010). There were parallel developments in India.

THE PARADOX IN REPRODUCTIVE POLICY IN INDIA—1950s TO 1970s

In this section, I describe the contradictory nature of the Indian government's biopolitical interventions over time. While the 1950s saw population control efforts, from the 1970s there was support from the state for the growing private industry in medicine and assisted reproduction.

India was the first country in the world to have a population policy, as early as 1952. Over time, the government implemented more targeted population policies (McBride 2012). In the 1970s the government began sterilization drives as part of its population control program. In 1975, during the period of National Emergency, Prime Minister Indira Gandhi's (1917–1984) son, Sanjay Gandhi (1946–1980), began forced sterilization of economically underprivileged and marginalized men. Described by many as a "gruesome campaign," around 6.2 million men in India were sterilized in a year. This number was said to be fifteen times more than the number of people sterilized during the Nazi regime. Historically, India has been known to have concentrated its population control efforts on the poor and the marginalized (Biswas 2014).

Subsequently, the development of technologies related to assisted conception, such as IVF, also saw increased focus on their use by women. The role of globalization, an increased focus on expanding technology in health programs, and an increasingly technocentric approach have been some of the key factors in the growth of assisted reproduction in India (Qadeer 2010).

HUMAN IN VITRO FERTILIZATION (IVF) IN INDIA

While the team in the UK was working toward the implementation of IVF, Subhas Mukhopadhyay (1931–1981) was working toward the development of the technique in his South Calcutta (Kolkata) apartment, with little equipment or financial support. Over time, he gained success but faced rebuke and much later posthumous recognition (Scientific Indians 2010; Mitra 1978). Mukhopadhyay (also referred to as Mukherjee or Mukerji) obtained a PhD in Reproductive Physiology in 1958 from the University of Calcutta. In 1967, he received another doctorate from the University of Edinburgh in Reproductive Endocrinology. Between 1967 and 1975, he questioned earlier methods and "played with the embryos and early stage foetus," presenting his work in Paris in 1977 (Dhawale 2014, 101).

Prabhat Agarwal was the eldest son of a wealthy family in Calcutta which moved from real estate and the stock market to trading in hosiery and garments. He and his partner Bela had difficulty conceiving in the first five years of their marriage (Mitra 1978). In 1974, Mukhopadhyay agreed to help the Agarwal couple provided they were discreet about the process (Mitra 1978). The need for discretion was felt by both Mukhopadhyay who did not want the family to talk about his "new method" and the Agarwals who were "very sensitive on the subject." The Agarwals reportedly refused an offer of a large amount of money from "a Japanese news agency to visit Japan for a month." Prabhat's father, Purushottam, was firm that "God did not give us this child to earn money." This was compared to the Browns who were criticized in the Indian press because it was reported they had "sold exclusive reporting rights of the birth of their baby to London's *Daily Mail*" (Mitra 1978, 37).

In 1978, Mukhopadhyay was the first in the world to successfully use a frozen and thawed embryo resulting in a birth. Unlike his counterparts in the United Kingdom, Mukhopadhyay and his team (which included a cryobiologist, Sunit Mukherjee, and a gynecologist, Saroj Kanti Bhattacharya) "used gonadotropins for ovarian stimulation, transvaginal colpotomy to harvest oocytes and cryopreservation of the human embryo" (Dhawale 2014, 102).

Kanupriya Agarwal (also known as Durga after the Hindu goddess) was born at Calcutta's (Kolkata's) Bellevue Nursing Home to Prabhat Kumar Agarwal and Bela Agarwal on October 3, 1978.[3] Prabhat requested the doctor to avoid publicity as he recognized that his partner was under a lot of mental strain (AAP-Reuter-AP 1978). Bhattacharya, heading the team of doctors responsible for Kanupriya's birth, remarked that if Bela had not belonged to a "conservative" family, he would have held a press conference "so that the world could have learnt from her about the experiment" (AAP-Reuter-AP 1978). This was the world's second and India's first birth conceived through IVF—just ten weeks after the birth of Louise Brown in the United Kingdom.

Mukhopadhyay's ten years of work on innovative techniques between 1967 and 1977 led to an approach to IVF different from Edwards and Steptoe in that he collected the ovum without the use of laparoscopy (Scientific Indians 2010). The method also differed from the British team in that they introduced the embryo into Lesley Brown's uterus seventy-two hours after the extraction of the ovum, while Mukhopadhyay's team kept the Agarwal embryo frozen for fifty-three complete days. This helped Bela Agarwal undergo a new ovulation cycle and come back to the same condition as at the time of ovum extraction (Mitra 1978, 36).

In November 1978, an expert committee appointed by the Government of West Bengal under the Medical Association convicted Mukhopadhyay of claiming to be "the architect of a human test-tube baby" known as Durga.

The committee declared that Mukhopadhyay had announced the reports to the media before clearance by government bureaucrats. It also said that Mukhopadhyay had used equipment and a refrigerator in his own home to conduct this experiment and that he had refused to "give in to government bureaucrats," thus attracting the jealousy of his peers. In December 1978, the same committee denounced his claims as "bogus" (Scientific Indians 2010). He was criticized for not reporting his research in peer-reviewed scientific journals. In 1980, there was a spate of incidents such as denial of leave to write up a detailed report of his results, social ostracism, bureaucratic negligence, reprimand, the denial of a passport to attend a meeting in Kyoto to discuss his work on IVF, and his transfer to the Institute of Ophthalmology as professor of electrophysiology. In the same year, Mukhopadhyay suffered a heart attack which has been attributed to the stress of these events (Scientific Indians 2010). Mukhopadhyay's colleague Sunit Mukherjee later reflected that while Edwards was eventually awarded the Nobel Prize, Mukhopadhyay's feat was "greeted with disbelief" and that the unbearable humiliation led Mukhopadhyay to end his life in 1981 (Jayaraman 2010). Bärnreuther highlights the importance of "space" and "place" in scientific knowledge production and calls Mukhopadhyay's innovation "out of place" because he conducted experiments outside "authorised institutions and recognised centers of innovation" (Bärnreuther 2016, 73).

In August 1986, Harsha Chawda, described as the first "scientifically documented" IVF baby, was born through the collaboration of doctors from the King Edward Memorial Hospital (KEM) and scientists from the Institute for Research in Reproduction (IRR) in Mumbai (Bharadwaj 2002).[4] Bharadwaj has traced the trajectory of ARTs in India through various moments in its growth. He unveils the politics of conception through a focus on the contested claims of various medical practitioners claiming the first baby conceived through IVF in India (Bharadwaj 2002). Bharadwaj argues that popular culture and print and electronic media, along with the mushrooming of IVF clinics in India, have "together popularized and normalized the idea of 'test-tube babies' in a country of more than a billion people" (Bharadwaj 2016b, 3).

Infertility management in India began with the provision of high-tech services through the public sector, which slowly moved to the private sector. Both infertility management and population control were the domains of the Indian government. Gradually, in the decades after the first IVF birth in India, biomedical research began to be funded by large private corporations. Over time, there was a movement to such services being offered by private fertility clinics and doctors (Bharadwaj 2000, 2002, 2016a, 2016b). The decade from the mid-1980s saw economic reforms leading to the privatization of health, an increased role of media, and a technocentric approach in selective healthcare such as fertility services.

ECONOMIC REFORMS

The period from 1987 to 1995 saw a host of economic reforms which influenced sectors like health and education. The opening up of the economy was one of the major factors that affected health policy, medical travel, and later reproductive travel. Public health experts in India have analyzed the political economy of health and of assisted reproduction in India. They have described increased commercialization and privatization of healthcare, especially with the liberalization of the economy which began in the early 1980s. The opening up of the economy in 1991 with the Structural Adjustment Programs (SAPs) of the Bretton Woods Institutions, however, slowed down growth, and brought about increased poverty and inflation. The SAPs were responsible for globalizing the Indian economy at a very fast pace and it is suggested that India only survived the crisis due to the sheer size of its economy. A major repercussion of the SAPs was a considerable reduction of government funding for healthcare programs and health infrastructure (Gangolli, Duggal, and Shukla 2005).

Imrana Qadeer has attributed the growth of assisted reproduction along with other technologies in India to multiple factors. These include an expanding medical market, the International Conference on Population Control and Development (ICPD)'s[5] promotion of ARTs in the name of choices for women, and the coming together of profit-generating promoters of medical marketization (Qadeer 2010). Amit Sengupta has written about the complexities of the growth of ARTs in a country like India where a large part of the population suffers from health problems like anemia, leprosy, and tuberculosis (Sengupta 2010). Yet the country also boasts a tertiary care sector that competes with institutions at an international level.

In the late 1970s, the Indian Council of Medical Research began to promote research in biomedicine and biotechnology. Over time, it decided to include ART Research in the "Family Welfare Programme and Tertiary Care Service Institutions in the Ninth Five Year Plan" (Qadeer 2010, 7). Sengupta adds that the neoliberal policies of 1991 created conditions for an already growing private sector in medical care. In addition, globalization has brought about an increase in consumerism in the medical sector. Profit maximization and growth expansion have been typical of corporate style functioning in medical care (Sengupta 2008).

Aditya Bharadwaj's extensive anthropological analysis of human IVF in India has revealed various factors in the growth of assisted reproduction. These factors include experts in the field leaving government clinics and moving to private practice for greater freedom and autonomy. A "media-medicine nexus" in the late 1980s and early 1990s, whereby the media gave credibility to claims of medical professionals working in particular state-run collaborations, contributed to the success of medical professionals. This was especially in relation to the contestation of "scientific facts" and "claims" regarding medical firsts. There was an oscillation in the 1980s and the 1990s from "awe and mistrust" to the "marvel of science" frame, resulting in popular science journalism assuming the form of an "institutional advertisement" for assisted reproduction. Other factors in the growth of assisted reproduction include economic liberalization in the country in 1991 and the incentivizing of infertility management, increased demand due to stigma around infertility, the growth of medical travel, and the promotion of ARTs, particularly in the private sector (Bharadwaj 2016a, 2000, 63, 2002). Sama Resource Center for Women and Health, a feminist action research group working on women's health-related issues, has enumerated reasons for the growth of commercial surrogacy in India. These include the initial lack of regulation, comparatively lower costs compared to developed countries, shorter waiting times, the large number of women available to engage in gestational surrogacy, and the state-of-the-art medical expertise and infrastructure (Sama 2012).

DUE RECOGNITION

Between 1978 and the early 2000s, the account of the history of IVF in India was reviewed and revised. As we have seen, Mukhopadhyay's contributions were at first discounted, with T. C. Anand (1936–2010) claiming the first "scientifically documented test tube baby" in Mumbai in 1986. In 1996, Anand Kumar, leader of the group and former director of IRR, gained access to Mukhopadhyay's papers and handwritten notes. Mukhopadhyay's colleague Sunit Mukherji helped Kumar access the documents. Kumar took a year to study them and wrote the first paper on Mukhopadhyay's achievements (Scientific Indians 2010; Kumar 1997).

In February 1997, at the Subhas Mukerji Memorial Oration at the third National Congress on Assisted Reproductive Technology and Advances in Infertility Management, held in Calcutta (Kolkata), Kumar appealed for posthumous recognition of Mukhopadhyay for the creation of India's first test-tube baby. A few months later, Kumar published an article recognizing Mukhopadhyay's invaluable contribution (Kumar 1997; Bharadwaj 2016a).

In 2002, the Indian Council for Medical Research (ICMR) recognized the contribution of Mukhopadhyay for the first time. In the following year, the committee accepted Mukhopadhyay's claim and rewrote the history of IVF. In 2004, IVF specialists across the country challenged the claim of Mukhopadhyay's achievement, but in 2005 the committee upheld the claim (Scientific Indians 2010). In 2007, an entry on Mukhopadhyay's life and work was published in the *Dictionary of Medical Biography* by the Wellcome

Trust Centre for the History of Medicine at University College London. The following April, Mukhopadhyay's achievement received the official stamp of approval by the Indian Council for Medical Research (Scientific Indians 2010). These controversies proceeded in the background of the growth in assisted reproductive services in India.

THE SCALE OF ASSISTED REPRODUCTION

There has been a steady and consistent growth in IVF services across the globe, especially since 2002 (Collins 2002; Jones et al. 2010). In 2002, IVF services were available in only one-quarter of the world's nations. These were mostly affluent nations, which accounted for more than 90 percent of the world's gross domestic product. By 2007, this had expanded to nearly a third of the world's nations. By 2010, more than half of the world's nations were on the verge of developing services related to IVF. Estimates show the existence of 4,000–4,500 IVF clinics globally with more than a quarter of the clinics in Japan and India (more than 600 clinics in Japan and more than 500 clinics in India) (Collins 2002; Jones et al. 2010). The mid-2000s also saw rapid growth and expansion of IVF services and clinics in the Middle East and Latin America. Despite Latin America ranking in the lowest quartile in the number of IVF clinics, nine individual Latin American countries were in the list of the top nations using IVF (Adamson 2009).

Due to the absence, until recently, of a national registry, there are no accurate statistics on the number of clinics, surrogate births, or births by assisted reproduction in India (Nadimpally, Marwah, and Shenoi 2011). In 2008, surrogacy was estimated to be a US$445 million industry in India (Indo-Asian News Service 2008). The Confederation of Indian Industry (CII) conducted a study in collaboration with McKinsey and Co and estimated that 150,000 medical travelers went to India in 2005 (Chinai and Goswami March 2007). In 2014, Manish Banker, president of the Indian Society for Assisted Reproduction (ISAR), said that the ART market in India was estimated to be worth $1 billion in the following three to five years and could double by 2018 (Pandit 2014). The International Medical Travel Journal suggested that there were at least 500 legal fertility clinics, out of which 350 offered surrogacy services (*International Medical Travel Journal* 2015).

CONTROVERSIES AROUND COMMERCIAL GESTATIONAL SURROGACY

As noted above, IVF and other elements of assisted reproduction allowed for the separation of fertilization, implantation, and gestation, making possible the use of gestational surrogacy and third-party provision of sperm and ova.

These forms of assisted reproduction became commercialized. A few transnational surrogacy cases were mired in ethico-legal battles which garnered media attention and led to moves for greater regulation.

There were a series of controversial cases which led the government to draft the surrogacy bill (to be discussed below) in its current shape. One was the case of "Baby Manji" Yamada. Manji was born in July 2008 at Akanksha Infertility Clinic in Anand, Gujarat. She was conceived from her father, Yamada Ikufumi's, sperm and an egg from an anonymous provider and carried by a gestational mother in India (Nair 2016). Before Manji's birth, the commissioning parents were divorced in Japan. Yamada as a single man could not adopt Manji due to adoption laws in both India and Japan (Mackie 2013, 2014b, 2014c). The Japanese legal system only recognizes the birth mother as the mother and the birth mother's husband as father, so that Manji could not obtain Japanese nationality. Although not legally banned, the Japan Society of Obstetrics and Gynecology prohibits its members from facilitating surrogacy. Indian laws at this stage did not address surrogacy directly. A birth certificate was refused to Manji due to uncertainty about the mother's name in the vital records register. When national advice was sought, a passport was refused. Lawyer Indira Jaisingh filed an appeal with the Indian government claiming Yamada to be Manji's father and arguing for Manji's right to live with her Japanese family and receive Japanese nationality. Manji's paternal grandmother, Yamada Emiko, filed a petition in Rajasthan High Court for "temporary custody as Manji's closest blood relative in India, until custody could be transferred to her son" (Points 2009, 5). Despite her genetic relationship with Yamada Ikufumi, Manji could not gain Japanese nationality from her father and was left illegitimate and stateless (Mackie 2013, 2014b, 2014c).

This landmark case raised questions regarding the kinship, parentage, and citizenship rights of babies born through cross-border assisted reproduction. Other cases that led to calls to regulate surrogacy included refusal by the German government to issue a visa to a baby born through surrogacy in Anand, Gujarat. The baby was later given Indian citizenship and the parents undertook adoption. In the Baby Dev case, Australian parents went to India for surrogacy but abandoned one of the twins born (a boy) while they took the girl away (Garg 2016; Nair 2016). Such controversies were the impetus for a host of draft regulations taking the form of bans and stricter enforceable laws. This was more visible especially after the year 2013 with the beginning of enforceable bans, as will be discussed below.

REGULATING ASSISTED REPRODUCTION

The years from 2005 witnessed numerous draft regulations, notifications, and guidelines and reflected the nature of the government's attempts to exert control over commercial transactions of gestational surrogacy in particular. This was primarily due to ethical and legal battles over some of the aforementioned controversies which had emerged during transactions related to assisted reproduction.

In 2005, the Ministry of Health and Family Welfare (MoHFW), Government of India (GoI), and ICMR released the first draft guidelines, namely, the National Guidelines for Accreditation, Supervision and Regulation of ART Clinics in India (Indian Council of Medical Research 2005). The Assisted Reproductive Technology (Regulation) Bill, 2008 (Ministry of Health and Family Welfare 2008), was followed by the Assisted Reproductive Technology (Regulation) Rules-2010 (Indian Council of Medical Research 2010b). In July 2012, a letter from the Government of India, Ministry of Home Affairs outlined that foreigners were visiting India on tourist visas to commission surrogacy and that it was not an appropriate visa category. Instead, they should obtain a medical visa to commission surrogacy (Sarma 2012).

In March and July 2013, there was a circular and then a letter from the Government of India, Ministry of Home Affairs regarding foreign nationals intending to visit India for commissioning surrogacy. In September of the same year, the ICMR released Steps for Registration under the National Registry of ART Clinics and Banks in India. In October 2013, a circular from Government of India, Ministry of Home Affairs referred to a letter from the Ministry of Home Affairs dated July 9, 2012, stating that the guidelines should be strictly followed, including all cases of commissioned surrogacy (Indian Council of Medical Research 2013; Srivastava 2013).

In January 2014 the Government of India, Ministry of Home Affairs released an Office Memorandum regarding a meeting to be held under the chairmanship of Joint Secretary (Foreigners) on January 28, 2014, to discuss procedures related to surrogacy. A list of such cases was to be given to the Foreigners Regional Registration Office (FRRO), Delhi, by the ART clinics. In addition, the letter mentioned that cases would be recognized only on receipt of a letter from the embassy of the foreign country stating that it did not prohibit surrogacy, and did not have specific laws on surrogacy, common law marriage, and cases involving cohabitation and legal action that could be used against ART clinics violating orders of the MHA.

In January 2014, ICMR announced a National Registry of Assisted Reproductive Technology (ART) Clinics and Banks in India. A few days later, Dr. R. S. Sharma from ICMR directed that surrogacy would be limited to Indian married couples only and not available to foreigners (Sharma 2014, 2015).

In 2015, the ICMR and the Government of India asserted that in order that a surrogate not be exploited, a medical visa could be granted to foreigners intending to visit India to commission surrogacy. Further, the foreign couple would be told that exit permission would be required from the FRRO, which would check whether they had a letter from the ART clinic. In November

2015, the Ministry of Home Affairs (Department of Health Research) issued directions regarding commissioning of surrogacy. The import of human embryos would be for research purposes only. Surrogacy clinics, ART clinics, or IVF clinics offering surrogacy or assisted reproductive services would not import human embryos for surrogacy. The government also issued "Other instructions regarding foreign nationals" (Sharma 2015; Government of India Ministry of Health and Family Welfare 2015; Chadha 2015).

In August 2016, the Department of Health Research released the draft Surrogacy Regulation Bill, 2016, banning commercial surrogacy and encouraging altruistic surrogacy from among female family members. It would ban commercial surrogacy for homosexuals, unmarried cohabiting couples, and heterosexual couples married for more than five years who have biological children. It would allow surrogacy for couples whose first child has a mental or terminal illness; genetic disorders like thalassemia, sickle-cell anemia, and hemophilia; or had died (Nair Sepember 8, 2016). It was introduced in the Lok Sabha (Lower House) in November 2016 and certain issues for consideration were raised (PRS Legislative Research November 2016).

Commentators argued that the Surrogacy Bill 2016 raised a host of concerns that needed to be "addressed through polemics" before a final shape would eventually emerge (Sengupta 2016, S18). Some of the biomedical concerns raised around the Surrogacy Bill 2016 included the near impossibility of declaring "infertility as a conclusive medical fact," the need for examination of age norms and the five-year wait after marriage before a couple could access surrogacy. Other concerns included couples with secondary infertility and a live biological child being forbidden from opting for surrogacy arrangements as well as the ambiguity in the definition of compensation to a surrogate mother in the form of "reasonable medical expenses" rather than the desirability of calculating "man-hour loss" as some argued (Ghosh 2016). Domestic altruistic surrogacy could potentially bring about exploitation and corruption and could even lead to relatives being generated for purposes of altruistic surrogacy or surrogates possibly being impregnated in the country and moved to jurisdictions with laxer laws (Malhotra 2016, S17).

The Parliamentary Standing Committee on Health and Family Welfare recognized that "surrogacy services should not be dismissed in paternalistic manner," and made a case for "reasonable compensation," but stated that surrogacy should not be allowed as a profession (Das 2017). The stigma attached to infertility could lead to women being at greater risk of domestic violence and abuse. Concern was expressed that the surrogate would develop emotional attachment to the child especially if she shared familial ties with intending parents. The Committee argued that "altruistic surrogacy only by close relatives" would "always be because of compulsion and coercion and not because of altruism" (Das 2017). The Committee also pointed out that the bill failed to recognize "the rights of live-in partners" and expressed concern about the five-year wait for surrogacy for those getting married in their thirties and forties (Das 2017). This was said to violate the right to reproductive autonomy. The report affirmed that surrogacy should not be indiscriminately extended to foreign nationals (Das 2017).

The Surrogacy Regulation Bill 2016 was passed by the Lok Sabha (Lower House) in December 2018 (Singh 2019). The legislation in its final form did not address the concerns outlined above. Under the new legislation, only altruistic (i.e., noncommercial) surrogacy is allowed. The intending parents can only cover medical costs and should take out medical insurance for the gestational mother (Banghra 2019). The intending parents should be a heterosexual married couple of Indian citizenship resident in India who have been legally married for at least five years. They need a doctor's certification that they are medically unfit to produce a child and should not have children of their own, unless their child is mentally or physically disabled or suffers from a life-threatening disorder with no permanent cure (Banghra 2019). The intending parents should be between the ages of 23 and 50 for women and between the ages of 26 and 55 for men. The child will be deemed to be the legal offspring of the intending couple. Surrogacy is not available to singles, non-heterosexual couples or unmarried cohabiting couples (Dey 2019). The person who provides gestational labor should be a close relative of one of the intending parents, be aged between 25 and 35, be married (or previously married), and have at least one child. The gestational surrogate may not be the provider of ova (Banghra 2019). The legislation allows for regulation in the form of a National Surrogacy Board at national level and state surrogacy boards at local level (Dey 2019; Rai 2018).

CONCLUSION

The history of in vitro fertilization in India is as old as in Britain, Australia, or the United States (Franklin 1997, 81). The history of IVF in India is not a linear narrative, but a rather convoluted one. India has seen major contributions by leading medical experts in the development of IVF. Over time, biopolitical interventions by the government have reiterated the role of the government in population control. The role of globalization and privatization in the mushrooming of fertility clinics and the nature of regulation itself speak of the commercial element in perpetuating social myths and aspects of identity related to infertility. In the past few years, the emphasis on restricting the use of reproductive services like IVF and surrogacy to particular kinds of groups and families reflects the state's role in creating and encouraging particular types of familial and kinship arrangements and disregarding others. Repronationalism, repronational histories, and repronational choreographies reveal the roles of different actors and institutions—from religion and media, to the state and family—which influence the use and access of technologies such as IVF in particular socio-politico-economic and cultural contexts. In addition, restrictions on access to reproductive services by those of non-Indian nationality affect the cross-border flow of clients in the global reproductive services industry, reflecting the transnational effects of biopolitical interventions at the national level (see Whittaker 2018; Marks, Mackie, and Ferber in this volume).

NOTES

1. Capacitation is "a final maturation process which spermatozoa undergo physiologically in the uterus and that is essential for the acquisition of fertilizing competence" (Johnson 2011, 254).

2. "This technique proved beneficial, in part due to the small abdominal incisions required to insert the laparoscope (a long telescope utilizing a light source) as well as allowing the physician to actually see inside the patient, affording the opportunity for more accurate diagnosis" (Danielson 2009, n.p.).

3. Prasad (1986) reports on a baby born in June 1986 in Bangalore (now Bengaluru) to H. T. and Nirupima Prakash. Their IVF treatment had been carried out in the United Kingdom, though, so this could not be claimed as a first for Indian science.

4. The National Institute for Research in Reproductive Health (NIRRH) was formerly known as the Institute for Research in Reproduction (IRR). The IRR was an amalgamation of The Contraceptive Testing Unit and the Reproductive Physiology Unit that came into being in 1970. In 1971, the Indian Council of Medical Research (ICMR hereafter) established a network of Contraceptive Testing Units that were later renamed the Human Reproduction Research Centres in the year 1980. The Indian Council of Medical Research (ICMR), earlier known as the Indian Research Fund Association (IRFA), had its first governing body meeting in November 1911 when the Scientific Advisory Board was constituted. In the year 1949, the IRFA was redesignated as the Indian Council of Medical Research. In 1969, the Division of Reproductive Biology and Fertility Control was created at the ICMR headquarters.

5. The First United Nations International Conference on Population and Development (ICPD) was held in Cairo in the year 1994. A twenty-year Program of Action was adopted by 179 countries.

WORKS CITED

AAP-Reuter-AP. 1978. "Father of Test-tube Baby Wanted Anonymity." *Sydney Morning Herald.*

Adamson, G. David. 2009. "Global Cultural and Socioeconomic Factors that Influence Access to Assisted Reproductive Technologies." *Women's Health* 5 (4): 351–58.

Bärnreuther, Sandra. 2016. "Innovations 'Out of Place': Controversies Over IVF Beginnings in India Between 1978 and 2005." *Medical Anthropology* 35 (1): 73–89.

Bavister, Barry D. 2002. "Early History of In Vitro Fertilization." *Reproduction* 124: 181–96.

Bhangra, Kulraj Singh. 2019. "India's Lower House Passes Bill Banning Commercial Surrogacy." *Bionews* 982 (January 14). Available at https://www.bionews.org.uk/page_140769 (Last accessed February 2, 2019).

Bharadwaj, Aditya. 2000. "How Some Indian Baby Makers are Made: Media Narratives and Assisted Conception in India." *Anthropology and Medicine* 7 (1): 63–78.

______. 2002. "Conception Politics: Medical Egos, Media Spotlights, and the Contest over Test-Tube Firsts in India." In *Infertility around the Globe: New Thinking on Childlessness, Gender, and Reproductive Technologies*, edited by Marcia C. Inhorn and Frank van Balen, 315–33. Berkeley, Los Angeles, London: University of California Press.

______. 2016a. "The Indian IVF Saga: A Contested History." *Reproductive BioMedicine and Society Online* 2 (Symposium: IVF- Global Histories): 54–61.

______. 2016b. *Conceptions: Infertility and Procreative Technologies in India*. New York: Berghahn Books.

Biswas, Soutik. 2014. "India's Dark History of Sterilisation." *BBC News*. http://www.bbc.com/news/world-asia-india-30040790 (Last accessed September 1, 2017).

Brinsden, Peter R. 2011. "The Evolution of ART." In *Principles and Practice of Fertility Preservation*, edited by Jacques Donnez and S. Samuel Kim, 1–10. Cambridge: Cambridge University Press.

Chadha, Sanjeev. November 4, 2015. *Commissioning of Surrogacy*. Ministry of Health and Family Welfare (Department of Health Research) Government of India.

Chang, Min Chueh. 1959. "Fertilization of Rabbit Ova In Vitro." *Nature* 184 (4684): 466–67.

Chinai, Rupa and Rahul Goswami. March 2007. "Medical Visas Mark Growth of India Medical Tourism." *Bulletin of the World Health Organization* 85 (3): 164–65.

Clarke, Gary N. 2006. "A.R.T. and History, 1678–1978." *Human Reproduction* 21 (7): 1645–50.

Cohen, J., A. Trounson, K. Dawson, H. Jones, J. Hazekamp, K. G. Nygren, and L. Hamberger. 2005. "The Early Days of IVF Outside the UK." *Human Reproduction Update* 11 (5): 439–59. doi: 10.1093/humupd/dmi016.

Collins, John A. 2002. "An International Survey of the Health Economics of IVF and ICSI." *Human Reproduction Update* 8 (3): 265–77.

Connelly, Matthew. 2008. *Fatal Misconception: The Struggle to Control World Population*. Cambridge, Massachusetts: The Belknap Press of Harvard University Press.

Danielson, Andrew. 2009. "Patrick Christopher Steptoe (1913–1988)." *Embryo Project Encyclopedia*. http://embryo.asu.edu/handle/10776/1759 (Last accessed July 31, 2018).

Das, Monalisa. 2017. "Surrogacy without Pay Unreasonable" Parl Committee Points Out Flaws with Draft Bill." *The News Minute*, August 12. https://www.thenewsminite.com/article/surrogacy-without-pay-unreasonable-parl-committee-points-out-flaws-draft-bill-66677 (Last accessed September 22, 2018).

Dey, Sushmi. 2018. "Lok Sabha Clears Bill Banning Commercial Surrogacy." *Times of India*, December 20. Available at https://timesofindia.indiatimes.com/india/lok-sabha-passes-surrogacy-regulation-bill-2016-which-bans-commercial-surrogacy/articleshow/67165408.cms (Last accessed February 2, 2019).

Dhawale, Avlikant J. 2014. "Dr. Subhas Mukherjee and India's First Test Tube Baby." *PharmaTutor* 2 (12): 99–106.

Foucault, Michel. 1978. *The History of Sexuality, Volume 1: An Introduction*. New York: Pantheon Books. Translated by Robert Hurley.

Franklin, Sarah. 1997. *Embodied Progress: A Cultural Account of Assisted Conception*. London and New York: Routledge.

______. 2016. "Changing Global Fertilities: A Third Demographic Transition?" *Reprosoc*, May 19. http://www.reprosoc.com/blog/2016/11/30/changing-global-fertilities-a-third-demographic-transition (Last accessed January 28, 2018).

Franklin, Sarah and Marcia C. Inhorn. 2016. "Introduction. Symposium: IVF-Global Histories." *Reproductive Biomedicine and Society Online* 2: 1–7.

Gallagher, James. 2013. "Obituary: Robert Edwards, Test-tube Baby Pioneer." *BBC News*, April 10. http://www.bbc.com/news/health-22095512 (Last accessed September 1, 2017).

Gangolli, Leena V., Ravi Duggal, and Abhay Shukla. 2005. *Review of Healthcare in India*. Mumbai: Centre for Inquiry into Health and Allied Themes.

Garg, Sanjeeb Ibu. 2016. "Understanding India's Complex Commercial Surrogacy Debate." *The Diplomat*, August 31. http://thediplomat.com/2016/08/understanding-indias-complex-commercial-surrogacy-debate/ (Last accessed January 28, 2018).

Ghosh, Debabrata. 2016. "Biomedical Considerations of the New Draft Surrogacy (Regulation) Bill, 2016." *Journal of Reproductive Health and Medicine* 2: S1–S2.

Government of India. 2018. The Surrogacy Regulation Bill, Bill No 257-C of 2016, Passed by Lok Sabha on December 19, 2018.

Government of India, Ministry of Health and Family Welfare. 2015. *Instructions Regarding Commissioning of Surrogacy*. New Delhi: Indian Council of Medical Research.

Indian Council Of Medical Research. 2010a. *The Assisted Reproductive Technologies (Regulation) Bill – 2010*. New Delhi: Government of India Ministry of Health and Family Welfare, Govt. of India.

———. 2010b. *The Assisted Reproductive Technologies (Regulation) Rules – 2010*. New Delhi: Government of India, Ministry of Health and Family Welfare.

———. *Enrolment Form for ART Clinics and Banks*. New Delhi: Indian Council of Medical Research.

———. 2013. *Steps for Registration under the National Registry for ART Clinics and Banks in India*. New Delhi: Indian Council of Medical Research.

Indian Council of Medical Research, National Academy of Medical Sciences. 2005. *National Guidelines for Accreditation, Supervision and Regulation of ART Clinics in India*. New Delhi: Government of India Ministry of Health and Family Welfare.

Indo-Asian News Service. 2008. "Surrogacy a $445 mn Business in India." *The Economic Times*. http://www.geneticsandsociety.org/article.php?id=4241 (Last accessed January 28, 2018).

International Medical Travel Journal. 2015. "India Introduces Legislation to Ban Surrogacy Tourism." December 7.

Johnson, Martin. 2011. "Robert Edwards: The Path to IVF." *Reproductive Biomedicine Online* 23 (2): 245–62.

Jones, Howard W. Jr., Ian Cooke, Roger Kempers, Peter Brinsden, and Doug Sanders. 2010. "International Federation of Fertility Societies Surveillance 2010: Preface." *Fertility and Sterility* 95 (2): 491.

Jayaraman, K. S. 2010. "Nobel to IVF Pioneer Revives Feelings of Loss." *Nature India*, October 10.

Kumar, T. C. Anand. April 1997. "Architect of India's First Test Tube Baby: Dr. Subhas Mukerji (January 16, 1931 to July 19, 1981)." *Current Science* 72 (7): 526–31.

Mackie, Vera. 2013. "Genders and Genetics: The Legal and Medical Regulation of Family Forms in Japan." *Australian Journal of Asian Law* 14 (1): 1–18.

———. 2014a. "Japan's Biopolitical Crisis." *International Feminist Journal of Politics* 16 (2): 278–96.

______. 2014b. "Birth Registration and the Right to Have Rights: The Changing Family and the Unchanging Koseki." In *Japan's Household Registration System and Citizenship: Koseki, Identification and Documentation*, edited by David Chapman and Karl J. Krogness, 201–20. London: Routledge.

______. 2014c. "Science, Society and the Sea of Fertility: New Reproductive Technologies in Japanese Popular Culture." *Japan Forum* 26 (4): 441–61.

Malhotra, Anil. 2016. "Surrogacy in India at Crossroads." *Journal of Reproductive Health and Medicine* 2: S16–S17.

McBride, Meredith. 2012. "History of Population Control in India." *Eye On Asia: Rights, Politics, And Goings-On In Asia.* https://humanrightsinasia.wordpress.com/2012/07/31/history-of-population-control-in-india/ (Last accessed September 1, 2017).

Ministry Of Health and Family Welfare, Government Of India. 2008. *The Assisted Reproductive Technology (Regulation) Bill, 2008*. New Delhi: Ministry of Health and Family Welfare.

Mitra, Sumit. 1978. "Test-tube Baby: Doctor's Dilemma." *India Today*, November 15.

Murthy, M. S. S. 2010. "Physiology or Medicine: Robert G. Edwards." *Science Reporter* (Nobel Prizes 2010): 30–32.

Nadimpally, Sarojini, Vrinda Marwah, and Anjali Shenoi. 2011. "Globalisation of Birth Markets: A Case Study of Assisted Reproductive Technologies in India." *Globalization and Health* 7 (27): 27.

Nair, Shalini. 2016. "From Abandonment to Abuse, 18 Cases that Helped Draft Surrogacy Bill." *The Indian Express*, September 8. http://indianexpress.com/article/india/india-news-india/surrogacy-bill-commercial-ban-indian-cases-sushma-swaraj-abandonment-abuse-girl-abortion-3019329/ (Last accessed September 29, 2018).

Pande, Amrita. 2011. "Transnational Commercial Surrogacy in India: Gifts for Global Sisters?" *Reproductive BioMedicine Online* 23 (5): 618–25.

Pandit, Virendra. February 18, 2014. "India's Fertility Market will be Worth Rs. 5,000 cr in Next Five Years." *The Hindu: Business Line*, February 18. https://www.thehindubusinessline.com/economy/indias-fertility-market-will-be-worth-rs-5000-cr-in-next-five-years/article23114098.ece (Last accessed September 22, 2018).

Points, Kari. 2009. *Commercial Surrogacy and Fertility Tourism in India*. Durham, NC: Kenan Institute of Ethics, Duke University.

Prasad, Srinivasa. 1986. "Test Tube Babies: Made in India." *India Today*, July 15.

PRS Legislative Research. November 2016. *Issues for Consideration: The Surrogacy (Regulation) Bill, 2016*. Edited by PRS Legislative Research.

Qadeer, Imrana. 2010. "New Reproductive Technologies and India's Transitional Health System." In *Making Babies: Birth Markets and Assisted Reproductive Technologies in India*, edited by Sandhya Srinivasan, 1–21. New Delhi: Zubaan and Sama.

Rai, Aasavri. 2018. "Cabinet Okays Moving Amendments to Surrogacy (Regulation) Bill, 2016." *Live Law.in*, March 22. http://www.livelaw.in/cabinet-okays-moving-amendments-surrogacy-regulation-bill-2016/ (Last accessed September 22, 2018).

Sama. 2012. *Birthing A Market: A Study on Commercial Surrogacy*. Sama Resource Group for Women and Health.

Sarma, G. V. V. July 9, 2012. *Notification Regarding Foreign Nationals Intending to Visit India for Commissioning Surrogacy*. New Delhi: Government of India Ministry of Home Affairs.

Scientific Indians. 2010. "The Untold Story Behind India's First Test Tube Baby." http://www.scientificindians.com/hall-of-fame/people/the-untold-story-behind-indias-first-test-tube-baby (Last accessed September 2, 2018).

Sengupta, Amit. 2008. "Medical Tourism in India: Winners and Losers." *Indian Journal of Medical Ethics* V (1) (January–March): 4–5.

———. 2010. "The Commerce in Assisted Reproductive Technologies." In *Making Babies: Birth Markets and Assisted Reproductive Technologies in India*, edited by Sandhya Srinivasan, 44–56. New Delhi: Zubaan and Sama.

Sengupta, Jayasree. 2016. "Opinions on the New Draft Surrogacy (Regulation) Bill, 2016 in India." *Journal of Reproductive Health and Medicine* 2: S18.

Sharma, R. S. 2014. *Announcement- National Registry of Assisted Reproductive Technology (ART) Clinics and Banks in India*. New Delhi: Indian Council of Medical Research.

———. 2015. *Regarding Foreigners Availing Surrogacy Services in India.* New Delhi: Indian Council of Medical Research.

Srivastava, Vikas. 2013. *Ministry of Home Affairs Letter.* New Delhi: Government of India, Ministry of Home Affairs.

Whittaker, Andrea. 2018. *International Surrogacy as Disruptive Industry in Southeast Asia.* New York: Rutgers University Press.

Yanagimachi, R. and M. C. Chang. 1963. "Fertilization of Hamster Eggs In Vitro." *Nature* 200 (4903): 281–82.

———. 1964. "In Vitro Fertilization of Golden Hamster Ova." *Journal of Experimental Zoology Part A: Ecological Genetics and Physiology* 156 (3): 361–75.

Chapter 3

"A Cloak and Dagger Situation"

Artificial Insemination, Secrecy and Openness in New Zealand, 1950s to Early 2000s

Jane Adams

Since 1990, donor openness has been a distinctive characteristic of New Zealand's experience of assisted reproductive technologies (ARTs), and an area where New Zealand, along with Sweden, has led the world (Daniels and Lewis 1996, 57). Fertility clinics in 1990 voluntarily adopted a policy of donor openness, which meant that gamete donors were required to be identifiable to their donor-conceived children. The Human Assisted Reproductive Technology Act 2004 (HART Act) later enshrined this openness policy into law, and the concept was embraced by politicians during the HART Act parliamentary debates (Part Three, HART Act). One politician, David Benson-Pope, in discussing New Zealand's "world-leading national information-keeping scheme" declared that donor openness in ART "reflected New Zealand's experiences of the consequences of closed adoption" and "the importance of knowledge about one's identity, family, and genetic heritage" (*New Zealand Parliamentary Debates* [NZPD] 2004, 621, 16837). Such acceptance of donor openness in ART was, however, a relatively recent development, and its longer history is one better characterized by secrecy.

In this chapter, I consider aspects of secrecy and openness in New Zealand's history of ART, focusing particularly on developments in artificial insemination (AI) from the mid-twentieth to early twenty-first century. The use of donor sperm in AI (AID) has been the major medical solution to male infertility for married couples for most of its recorded history. Just as AI's history is an area shrouded in secrecy and silences, male infertility has largely been an invisible area, relative to the greater attention paid to the treatment of female infertility by the medical profession and media. I will examine the medical practice of AI and its regulation, and consider the larger societal shifts that helped shape these changing responses to secrecy and openness in AI, drawing primarily upon published sources, including medical journals and textbooks, popular newspapers and magazines, legislation, government reports, and parliamentary debates.[1]

International studies have provided a useful backdrop for my discussion in this chapter. AI was and still is used as a medical practice to help infertile individuals and couples to form their families. Leading infertility historians Naomi Pfeffer, Elaine Tyler May, and Margaret Marsh and Wanda Ronner's respective scholarship provides helpful insights into broader historical developments in infertility and ART, including AI, in the United Kingdom and United States (Pfeffer 1993; May 1997; Marsh and Ronner 1996). Wendy Mitchinson's history of the Canadian medical profession's responses to infertility prior to 1950 provides useful discussion about doctors' relative neglect and reticence in treating their male infertility patients (Mitchinson 1993). Antje Kampf's study of male infertility medicine in 1950s and 1960s Germany similarly contains insights relevant to the New Zealand context. Kampf has discussed her problems in accessing the "'hidden' story of male infertility" in Germany, and this has been an area that I too have found difficult to access (Kampf 2014, 154). Gayle Davis's essay on medical responses to the infertile patient in mid-twentieth-century Scotland focused upon the Feversham Committee's inquiry into AI, which I discuss in this chapter (Davis 2013). In New Zealand, Paul Reynolds has explored contemporary Māori men's experiences of fertility, infertility, and sexuality. He suggests that fertility and infertility services are centered on females, and there is "a need to address the gap in service and voice of men's role, place and needs" (Reynolds 2012, 314–15). Lynne Batty has considered the development of social policy in assisted reproductive technologies in New Zealand, including AI. This policy had developed, she concluded, in a "fragmented, unplanned and reactive way" and Māori perspectives were ignored and marginalized during the policy debates (Batty 2002, 4). Anne Else has examined New Zealand's history of closed stranger adoption (Else 1991), a subject closely interconnected, as I will show, to medico-legal responses to AI. Linda Bryder has discussed the medical history of AI at National Women's Hospital (NWH) in Auckland, from the 1970s and 1980s (Bryder 2014, 111–12). In this chapter, I will build upon Bryder's work by discussing the earlier medico-legal history of AI in New Zealand, thus providing a new contribution to the international scholarship. Mark Henaghan, Ken Daniels, and John Caldwell's legal essay provides a particularly good overview of the complex myriad of government policy papers, ethics committees, professional self-regulation initiatives, and legislation in the area of ART since the 1980s (Henaghan, Daniels, and Caldwell 2007).[2] Since the early 1980s, social worker and scholar Ken Daniels's large body of research into donor conception and secrecy and openness has made a significant contribution to ART scholarship (e.g., Daniels 2004), and I have drawn upon Daniels's work in this chapter.

EARLY AI HISTORY, PRE-1950s

AI, although considered a relatively simple medical procedure, has attracted controversy and secrecy throughout most of its documented history. The medical practice of AI using the husband's sperm (AIH) was first performed by Dr. John Hunter (1728–1793) in England in the late eighteenth century and by gynecologist J. Marion Sims (1813–1883) in the United States in 1866 (May 1997, 67). In 1884, Dr. Robert William Pancoast (1835–1897) started performing AID in the United States in circumstances of great secrecy—at least from the female patient's perspective. The female patient in his first case was apparently administered chloroform before the procedure was carried out; they used the sperm of one of his medical students in attendance; and she was not informed that the child she conceived was not genetically related to her partner. In the early twentieth century, the idea of introducing a sperm donor into the process of reproduction was one "intriguing to eugenicists and appalling to moralists" (May 1997, 67). AID was promoted as a strategy for eugenic purposes in countries such as the United States, France, Australia, and the United Kingdom in the interwar period. US gynecologist Robert Latou Dickinson (1861–1950), an ally of the birth control advocate Margaret Sanger (1879–1966), was one of the first doctors to provide an AID service and was at the forefront of the "efflorescence of research into different aspects of human sexuality and reproduction" in the interwar period (Pfeffer 1993, 53). While eugenics-minded organizations in New Zealand were similarly concerned with promoting motherhood and Pākeha "race improvement" in the interwar period, I have not discovered any sources that promoted human AID solely for eugenic purposes.[3]

AI was first used in New Zealand's livestock programs from the 1930s, on an experimental basis, and on a commercial basis from the late 1940s (Dalton and Rumble 1985, 5 and 19). Artificial insemination first entered New Zealand's statute books under the Sharemilking Agreements Act 1937. Despite AI's economic value to farmers, its necessary association with reproduction led to some unease among farmers, just as in the human AI context (Dalton and Rumble 1985, 31). Similarly, religious responses toward AI in the New Zealand press from the 1930s were decidedly negative. The Catholic Church was the most vocal in its opposition to the practice. The Church considered AI unnatural, as it separated the act of sexual intercourse within marriage from conception. AI also required the semen provider to masturbate, which was a sin (*Press* 1945).

AI DEVELOPMENTS, 1950s AND 1960s

Medical commentators in New Zealand first began mentioning AI in their published discussions of infertility in the 1950s, and it was being used by an unknown number of New Zealand's doctors (See Mears 1950). This development formed part of their growing interest in the treatment of infertility and the establishment of the hospital-based infertility clinics, with the first one opening within Auckland's National Women's Hospital in 1950 (Bryder 2014, 33). Where New Zealand doctors wrote about AI in medical journals and texts, they did so guardedly and none acknowledged using AI as part of their own infertility practices. One doctor, while stating that AIH posed "few objections," cautioned doctors to be aware of AID's "genetical considerations" and the "legal and moral position before undertaking anything so highly controversial" (Mears 1950, 384). These "genetical considerations" refer to growing AID moral panics over "mutant genes" during the 1940s (Pfeffer 1993, 121). Some commentators feared that the chances of incestuous relationships—leading to children with "mutant genes"—was a statistical possibility, in theory, in a small country of New Zealand's size, which was about 2 million at this time.

Marriage was an essential prerequisite for couples seeking infertility services, such as AI, from doctors in the 1950s (Adams 2016). The possible involvement of a donor—another adult male—in the AI process was another major reason for legal scrutiny of AI, as it raised moral and legal concerns about the nature of the sacrosanct marriage relationship, and specifically whether using AI could constitute adultery under divorce laws (Northey 1958, 531). This was not a concern unique to New Zealand, as it was contentious elsewhere from the 1940s onward, and a number of judicial decisions and government inquiries in the United Kingdom, Canada, the United States, and Australia examined that very issue ("Recommendation 2(a). Human Artificial Insemination: Feversham Committee's Report," 1960, 379). In the United Kingdom, the Feversham Committee, which convened in 1958, recommended that AID be strongly discouraged. It made it an offense for anyone other than a doctor to carry out this procedure ("Human Artificial Insemination: Feversham Committee's Report," 1960, 379–80). The Committee recommended that "acceptance by a wife of AID without the consent of her husband should be made a new ground for divorce" ("Recommendation 2(a). Human Artificial Insemination: Feversham Committee's Report," 1960, 379). The UK Parliament did not enact this recommendation when its divorce laws were amended in 1969. When New Zealand's Parliament amended its divorce laws, however, section 21(1)(b) of the Matrimonial Proceedings Act 1963 stated: "It will be a ground for divorce that the wife has without her husband's consent, been artificially inseminated with the seed of another man."

Contemporary published discussions provide few clues as to why New Zealand's politicians considered this curious divorce ground necessary, particularly given the widespread secrecy surrounding AI practice, and the likelihood that only a "few practitioners" were prepared to carry it out due to legal and ethical concerns (Northey 1958, 533). I would speculate, however, that broader societal concerns about women's sexual behavior in early 1960s New Zealand may have influenced Parliament. The introduction of the oral contraceptive pill in 1961 had generated both excitement and concerns about the "life-changing promises" it held out for married women, who could now plan their lives to include a career and children—and possibly extramarital relationships (Brookes 2016, 330). Women's greater independence was an unsettling prospect for many men. Married women were moving into the workforce in growing numbers, and by 1966, nearly 20 percent of married Pākehā women were in the paid workforce, compared to 8 percent in 1945 (Mein Smith 2012, 200). AID was a practice that women in infertile marriages sought out in order to become mothers, whereas the contraceptive pill helped women to avoid motherhood and enjoy greater sexual freedom, inside and outside of marriage. On the face of it, the two fertility issues were not directly connected. The necessary involvement of male semen donors in AID, though, was associated with broader societal concerns about the potential for greater sexual freedoms enjoyed by women. The sperm donor was considered by many as a third party intruding into marriage and therefore committing adultery. The government's divorce law reforms arguably formed part of broader efforts to "advocate domesticity" in the early 1960s and to curb women's freedoms (Mein Smith 2012, 201).

AID posed other legal concerns. These included the legitimacy of the donor-conceived child. Under New Zealand's common law system, inherited from the United Kingdom, the semen donor was the child's legal father, and the child was illegitimate (Henaghan 2007, 34). This then had potential repercussions under inheritance laws, if the child's paternity was later questioned (Northey 1958, 533). Legal privilege was not available to protect doctors from liability where questions of the child's legitimacy were raised; and a husband could attempt to compel a doctor to give evidence of the AI procedure (Northey 1958, 532–33). Doctors were advised to destroy their AI records, as this was the only way to effectively protect both themselves from liability and the anonymity of the sperm donor (Northey 1958). Such advice further added to the secrecy surrounding the practice.

ESTABLISHMENT OF AI CLINICS AND CHANGING ADOPTION PRACTICES, 1970s

During the 1970s, AI became relatively more visible in New Zealand. The use of fresh semen in AID practice had been problematic for doctors, as they had faced issues concerning donor recruitment and the timing of insemination. The development of "sperm banks" (sperm cryopreservation) opened up new possibilities. Following trends in AI developments in Australia (Cox 1991, 258; Hill 1970), New Zealand's first hospital-based AI clinic was established in Auckland in 1972, by Dennis Bonham, head of National Women's Hospital Postgraduate School of Obstetrics and Gynaecology (Bryder 2014, 111). The clinic encountered opposition for "religious reasons" and Bonham—usually a vocal advocate of infertility services—did not attempt to publicize it (Bryder 2014, 111). A second clinic was soon opened in Christchurch, in New Zealand's South Island ("Controlled Artificial Insemination," 1978, 16). During this decade, patient demand for AI continued to grow, despite the unresolved legal issues associated with the practice. Why was this the case?

Developments in adoption practice and changing family forms in broader society were two significant factors driving this demand. A system of closed stranger adoption had been introduced in New Zealand law, via the Adoption Act 1955, and it quickly became a popular, nonmedical solution to infertility, enabling childless couples to create their own nuclear families. All legal ties were severed with the child's biological parents, which enabled the fact of the adoption to be concealed from the wider community. By the 1970s, however, social mores were changing rapidly in New Zealand and in particular the "advent of women's liberation spawned powerful forces" (Brookes 2016, 351–52). The Status of Children Act 1969 had removed the legal distinction between children born in and out of wedlock and made all children of equal status. Legislation passed in the late 1960s made it easier, in theory, for single mothers to obtain maintenance payments from fathers; removed the legal distinction between children born in and out of wedlock; and made all children of equal status.[4] New Zealand's general marriage rate peaked in 1971 and de facto relationships were increasing. Single women supporting children were prominent among those vocal in requesting state support and, by 1973, babies were increasingly staying with their single mothers rather than going to strangers (childless couples) for adoption (Brookes 2016, 352). In 1973, the government's introduction of the Domestic Purposes Benefit for single mothers allowed women to keep their children, causing a so-called shortage of babies for adoption (Else 1991, 159). By 1979 the number of babies and children available for closed stranger adoption was at its lowest point since the system was first introduced in 1955, and only a third of all adoptions were stranger adoptions (Else 1991, 171). Childless couples, unable to become parents via adoption, were increasingly turning their attention to medical solutions for infertility such as AID.

IVF DEVELOPMENTS AND REGULATORY DEBATES, 1980s

In vitro fertilization (IVF), another form of ART, then created new medical possibilities for childless couples. From the late 1970s IVF developments in the United Kingdom and in Melbourne, Australia—both world leaders in this area—were regularly reported in New Zealand and generated ongoing public discussion about whether IVF might be used to treat infertile couples in New Zealand (Adams 2017, 113). New Zealand couples traveled to Melbourne at their own expense to participate in IVF programs from the early 1980s onward and comprised the largest group of medical travelers on the waiting list (Ray 1983). In undertaking this form of reproductive travel, they were following in the footsteps of New Zealand women who had flown to Australia for abortions in the late 1970s, because of legal restrictions placed on abortion (Brookes 2016, 370–71).[5]

New Zealand's newspapers and mainstream magazines regularly and sympathetically reported on IVF travel (Adams 2017, 119). IVF was depicted positively as a way for married couples to become parents. The possibility of involving third-party donors in IVF, or in AI, though, rarely formed part of these initial discussions. New Zealand's first "test-tube" baby—conceived as a result of the parents' participation in the Royal Women's Hospital IVF program in Melbourne—was born in Christchurch in March 1983, followed a few months later by twins conceived as part of the same program (*Press* 1983, 1). The pending births of New Zealand's first "homegrown" IVF babies were announced in December 1983, following the establishment of New Zealand's first IVF program at National Women's Hospital, led by Dr. Freddie Graham (Bryder 2014, 112–16).

From the outset, Graham's team at National Women's Hospital deliberately adopted what they called a "conservative approach" to IVF (Graham et al. 1985, 180). Looking to overseas debates about IVF, such as in Melbourne, they anticipated that the introduction of IVF would be controversial among some segments of society.[6] Aiming to circumvent objections to IVF, they avoided using particular techniques which had attracted legal and ethical concerns in other countries, such as the use of donor sperm, eggs, or embryos in IVF. Graham emphasized, in March 1984, that he wanted people to feel reassured about what the IVF team were doing and that they were "playing it very safe" and "being ultra-conservative" (*New Zealand Truth* 19 June,

1984). The program was initially restricted to married couples, as a further way of appeasing critics.

IVF developments soon focused public attention on other approaches to infertility, particularly AI. Hospital-based AID programs had continued to expand in New Zealand in the 1980s due to ongoing patient demand. AID was, in theory, a more accessible infertility procedure than IVF. Until 1987, IVF was only available in one New Zealand city (Auckland), treating fifty couples per year, and the publicly funded Auckland program had long waiting lists for treatment (Bryder 2014, 114). New Zealand couples continued to travel to Australia for IVF treatment throughout the 1980s and into the 1990s, although their access rights, as non-Australians, to Australian healthcare services were sometimes contentious (National Bioethics Consultative Committee and Australian Health Ministers' Conference 1991, 26). By 1985, though, AI schemes were operating in all of New Zealand's main centers as well as in other smaller centers (Law Reform Division 1985).

Maintaining secrecy was an integral part of all AI schemes in the early to mid-1980s. All four major schemes attempted to match the "physical characteristics" of the husband and donor. The educational backgrounds of both men were considered in the Auckland, Wellington, and Christchurch programs (Law Reform Division 1985). The donor's identity was kept confidential, although biological data on the donor was collected and could be made available to the infertility patients. Couples in the Auckland AI program were, in its first decade of operation, advised to "go home, have sex and pretend it was theirs" after undergoing AID (Watkin 1998). This was less controversial advice than the practice of combining the donor's sperm and husband's sperm prior to insemination (known as AIC). Before the 1980s, AIC was used in the Auckland AI program, and probably other ones, as a way of further protecting the donor from any legal responsibility for the child.[7] Couples were advised to tell no one of their AID treatment, not even the child (Watkin 1998). Until 1984, donor registers enabling future tracing by donor-conceived adults were not kept (Watkin 1998). The early AI program was, as a doctor later reflected, a "cloak and dagger situation," due to the great secrecy surrounding it (Watkin 1998).

These deceptions in AI practice had strong parallels with closed stranger adoption practice in New Zealand from the 1950s, whereby adoption facilitators had attempted to match the physical characteristics of the adopted child with his or her adoptive parents in order to preserve secrecy (Else 1991, 70). Secrecy was evident in AI practice in the United States too in the 1970s and 1980s, where contemporary surveys showed that the "overwhelming majority" of doctors who performed AID agreed that "such a choice should remain a secret decision within the marriage" (Marsh and Ronner 1996, 228). One group of doctors surveyed said that, without exception, patients did not want to recall the experience. A prominent practitioner observed that "not even the grandparents should know" (Marsh and Ronner 1996, 228).

AI came under renewed legal scrutiny as a result of IVF discussions. The introduction of "no-fault divorce" in 1980, whereby the spouse filing for divorce did not have to show wrongdoing on the other spouse's part, now made the earlier question of whether AID was adultery irrelevant (O'Neill 1983, 2). Instead, commentators urged that action was needed to address the uncertain legal position of donor-conceived children. They wanted the law changed to make it clear that children conceived via AID were legally recognized as the children of the mother's husband ("the social father") rather than the biological father, the anonymous sperm donor. In 1984 former attorney-general Jim McLay acknowledged that there could well be "some hundreds of children alive today in New Zealand who were born as a result of AID procedures" (McLay 1984, 50). Sperm donation in AID remained the only form of donor conception being used in New Zealand's infertility clinics in the 1980s, as an egg donation program had not been established.[8] As a result, politico-legal discussions remained focused upon the role of fathers in families, and the prevalent assumption was that an anonymous sperm donor would want no ongoing involvement in the donor-conceived child's life (Adams 2017, 166).

In 1984—the year that New Zealand's first "IVF baby" was born—a consortium of New Zealand's leading medico-legal organizations requested that the government appoint a standing committee to consider the pressing "legal, social and moral issues" arising from IVF, AID, and related bioethical problems (Brinkman et al. 1985).[9] Responding to these concerns, the government took initial action in 1985 with its discussion paper, *New Birth Technologies*, which examined IVF, AI, and surrogate motherhood (Law Reform Division 1985). *New Birth Technologies* drew heavily upon the Warnock Committee report produced in the United Kingdom in 1984 and the Waller Committee report produced in Victoria, Australia, in 1983, but it "did not explore the issue in anything like the depth of those or many other overseas reports" (Henaghan, Daniels, and Caldwell 2007, 226).[10] Māori perspectives on the use of ART were notably absent from these politico-legal discussions, just as they were absent from other scholarly and mainstream publications about infertility and ART in the 1980s (Adams 2017, 149).

Minister of Justice Geoffrey Palmer, in introducing the *New Birth Technologies* discussion paper, observed that Victoria and the United Kingdom had "led the world in IVF techniques" and their government-appointed committees had "spent two years weighing the evidence before recommending courses of action," and for that reason, a "hasty reaction" from the New Zealand government was "neither possible nor desirable" (Law Reform Division, 7). AI was then—in effect—the only area on which Parliament took action the following year, when the Status of Children Amendment (SOCA) Bill was introduced and debated in 1986–1987. The SOCA Bill's stated purpose was to address the "status of persons conceived as a result of certain medical procedures," which suggests that the donor-conceived child was its focus (Status of Children Amendment Act 1987, No. 185).[11] The debates leading up to its eventual passing in 1987 clearly demonstrate Parliament's preoccupation with the *adult* relationships in AID rather than the children (donors were still not being used in IVF treatment). A general consensus emerged that married couples should be permitted to access ART treatments, on the premise that enabling infertile married—and implicitly heterosexual—couples to create families would help to strengthen and preserve the institution of marriage and the two-parent nuclear family model. Allowing heterosexual de facto couples to access infertility services attracted no such consensus in Parliament and several politicians were critical of the SOCA Bill's recognition of de facto couples, alongside married ones, and expressed concerns that the SOCA Bill would encourage such relationships (NZPD, 1986, 473, 3872). The possibility that same-sex couples might seek access to ART was given no serious attention in Parliament, with only one MP raising this prospect as "an undesirable consequence" of broadening access rights to ART (NZPD, 1987, 482, 10534–5).[12]

Parliament's commitment to the traditional two-parent nuclear family was affirmed in the final legislation, the Status of Children Amendment Act 1987. This Act excluded the biological parent (the gamete donor) from legal parenthood, just as the Adoption Act 1955 had extinguished the rights of biological parents to legal parenthood. This ongoing preference for the nuclear family form in the legislation failed to reflect ongoing socio-legal changes well underway in New Zealand society. In 1985 Parliament had enabled adult adoptees to access information about their biological parents (Adult Adoption Information Act 1985), in response to concerns that the secrecy surrounding closed stranger adoptions had been harmful. Family forms had been rapidly changing from the 1970s onward, shifting from the nuclear family to "an increasingly wide range of family forms" (Pool, Dharmalingam, and Sceats 2007, 218). The number of adults living in de facto relationships continued to increase steadily, and between 1981 and 1991, there was an increase of 84 percent in de facto relationships for those aged between twenty and thirty-nine years (Henaghan 2007, 8). Marriage rates had fallen by a third from the early 1970s to the mid-1980s, and the introduction of no-fault divorce helped divorce rates to rise (Carlyon and Morrow 2013, 235). Sole parent households had also continued to increase, from 5.1 percent in 1976 to 9.3 percent by 1991 (Pool, Dharmalingam, and Sceats 2007, 250). By the late 1980s, the nuclear family comprised just over a third of New Zealand families (Carlyon and Morrow 2013, 235).

These wider socio-legal changes were not limited to heterosexual couples. The Homosexual Law Reform Bill, introduced to Parliament in 1985, faced fierce opposition from conservative groups (Brookes 2016, 413; Brickell 2009, 480–82). The first part of the Bill, which decriminalized homosexuality, passed in the same month that the SOCA Bill was introduced to Parliament. While a (slim) majority of politicians agreed that homosexual men should not face criminal sanctions (lesbian women's relationships had never been criminalized), the possibility that same-sex couples might wish to access ART in order to become parents was clearly something these same politicians did not seriously anticipate during the SOCA Bill debates. Infertility treatments remained very much the prerogative of married heterosexual couples in 1980s New Zealand, and secrecy in donor conception remained the norm.

DONOR OPENNESS, 1990s–2004

Responses to donor conception and access rights to ART underwent a significant transformation in the 1990s. New Zealand fertility clinics' voluntary adoption of a donor openness policy from 1990—which meant that donors and recipient parents were advised to be open about genetic origins—was one important factor that contributed to this shift. Policy and legal developments in the previous decade helped to bring about this change. From the early 1980s, a more open style of adoptions had become the norm, with birth and adoptive parents meeting each other prior to the adoption and sometimes maintaining contact (Dalley 1998, 336–42). Social workers' experiences in the area of open adoption practices then informed their approaches toward donor conception (Adams 2017, 152). Social workers such as Ken Daniels and Joi Ellis played a prominent public role in advocating for a donor openness policy. A number of influential studies showed that a child's right to their genetic heritage was ignored by secrecy in AID programs (Adair and Rogan 1998).[13] The Status of Children Amendment Act 1987 had removed any legal liability to the gamete donor for the donor-conceived child, and so male donors no longer faced the possibility of paternity suits, child support obligations, and succession claims.

Māori perspectives on donor conception and ART increasingly featured in public discussions in the 1990s—or rather, commentators recognized the need for greater consultation and research in this area. The importance of *whakapapa* (knowing your ancestry) to Māori became recognized as central to their responses to using ART—and donor secrecy was completely at odds with this value (Glover 2007; Mead 2003). The Māori practice of *whāngai*, whereby Māori children were brought up within the extended family by people (sometimes infertile couples) who were not their biological parents, did not have the secrecy attached to it that Pākeha closed stranger adoption practices did (Smith 2012). Māori health researcher Dr. Paparangi Reid coauthored a leading Ministerial Committee report on ART, *Assisted Human Reproduction*, which demonstrated greater awareness of Māori views compared to previous government reports such as *New Birth Technologies* (Ministerial Committee on Assisted Reproductive Technologies 1994). Its guiding principles referred to the Treaty of Waitangi, New Zealand's founding document on the relations between Māori and Pākehā, stating it was vital that the development of ART in New Zealand recognized and protected "the rights and responsibilities of Treaty partners" (Ministerial Committee on Assisted Reproductive Technologies 1994, 30). This principle was later enshrined in the HART Act 2004 (under section 4(f)).

Medicolegal developments in ART in the 1990s helped to further transform responses toward traditional family forms and parenting (Ministerial Committee on Assisted Reproductive Technologies 1994, 54–55). Lesbians continued to publicly challenge what were seen as traditional approaches toward marriage and parenting and, following the introduction of the Human Rights Act 1993,[14] this now extended to well-publicized legal efforts to gain access to the fertility clinics' AID programs.[15]

The Intra-Cytoplasmic Sperm Injection, a variation on the original IVF procedure (ICSI-IVF) whereby a single sperm was injected into the cytoplasm (center) of the human egg, was a suitable treatment for men diagnosed with low sperm counts, and was first used by New Zealand's fertility clinics in 1994 (Adams 2017, 200). ICSI-IVF enabled infertile heterosexual couples to use the male partner's sperm, rather than donor sperm. Within a couple of years, heterosexual couples' requests for donor sperm and usage of AID had dramatically decreased (Adams 2017, 201). AID, which had been the major medical solution for male infertility in the 1980s, was instead more frequently used to help lesbian and single women form their families from the mid-1990s onward (Adams 2017, 221).

The profile and role of donors also came under scrutiny in other, interrelated ways in the 1990s. The establishment of New Zealand's first egg donor program in 1991 generated debate about whether or not egg donation within families should be permitted. This, in turn, helped challenge prevalent ideas about maintaining donor anonymity (Adams 2017, 186). Leading AID scholar Ken Daniels had shown that semen donors, rather than being disinterested parties, which was the popular perception, were sometimes interested in finding out about their donor-conceived children (Daniels 1987, 177). These changes all had flow-on implications for acceptance of donor openness.

ART Bills were introduced to Parliament in 1996 and 1997, and the HART Act finally passed in 2004. It formed part of a broad package of socio-legal reforms introduced by Helen Clark's Labour-Alliance government from 1999 onward. Politicians, in debating this legislation, drew attention to the new "ethos of openness" in New Zealand society (NZPD, 2004, 104, 15907), as reflected in their acceptance of donor openness in ART. Many politicians discussed the importance of a donor-conceived child knowing his or her origins, drawing analogies with New Zealand's adoption history and the damaging effects of secrecy (NZPD, 1998, 573, 13234–5). Some identified the value Māori placed on donor openness as a distinctive factor in New Zealand's experience of ART, and one which differentiated it from other countries (NZPD, 1997, 482, 1220; NZPD, 2004, 104, 15907).[16] They did not, however, engage in fuller discussions about Māori responses toward donor conception at this time. The country's relatively small size was considered a major factor supporting the need for donor openness, with some MPs, such as Sue Kedgley, expressing concern about the risk of incestuous relationships being formed by children who were not aware of their donor origins (NZPD, 2004, 104, 15934).

Tracking medicolegal responses to AI over half a century allows us to appreciate the sheer extent of the transformation in practices and attitudes in the broader area of family formation and parenthood. In the middle of the twentieth century, AI was a secretive, shameful practice. Through its legal association with adultery and divorce, it was perceived that it could potentially destroy families. By the 1980s, AI was becoming a more established medical practice, and politicians responded to it positively, acknowledging its ability to allow infertile married couples to become parents—and in doing so, to possibly "save" troubled marriages. Donor secrecy was still assumed, however, as the two-parent heterosexual family remained the ideal, and concurrent developments in adoption and homosexual law reform were not considered. Within ten years, donor openness in ART—promoted by a resurgence in Māori culture, human rights developments, open adoption practices, egg donation programs, and greater visibility of same-sex couples as parents—had become the new norm. What had once been a marital secret for heterosexual parents within a nuclear family was now a more open practice accessible to a far wider range of adults, and subject to official record-keeping and regulations.

NOTES

1. I draw upon additional types of medico-legal sources in my doctoral dissertation, such as case law and medical students' dissertations (Adams 2017).

2. I only discuss the major politico-legal developments—see Henaghan, Daniels and Caldwell's (2007) essay for fuller coverage.

3. "Pākehā" is a Māori-language term to describe New Zealanders of European descent. "Race improvement" formed part of the focus of positive eugenics

advocates. Martin Richards has considered sex educator and eugenist Marion Piddington's efforts in Australia, following the First World War, to promote AID as a form of "scientific motherhood" for use by war widows and single women (Richards 2008).

4. These statutes were the Domestic Proceedings Act 1968 and Legal Aid Act 1969 (Else 1991, 161).

5. Abortion was a controversial area of reproductive health in twentieth-century New Zealand, particularly in the 1970s when it was the subject of a government inquiry. For discussion, see Brookes (2016, 367–71).

6. For discussion about IVF controversies in Melbourne, see, for example, Leeton (2013) and Kannegiesser (1988).

7. The rationale for using AIC was because it made it difficult to determine who was the biological father. The husband could avoid committing perjury when he was named as the child's father on the birth certificate. Northey (1958) describes AIC in his article. Another practice of using two separate donors (women usually had two or three inseminations per procedure) had also ceased by the late 1970s (Watkin 1998).

8. For discussion about why New Zealand's egg donor program was delayed, see Adams (2017, 183–87).

9. The organizations were the Royal Society of New Zealand, the New Zealand Law Society, the Medical Council of New Zealand, the Medical Research Council of New Zealand, and the Medical Association of New Zealand.

10. Dame Mary Warnock chaired the sixteen-person committee (Committee of the Inquiry into Human Fertilisation and Embryology and M. Warnock 1984). The Waller Committee was a nine-person committee to consider the social, ethical, and legal issues arising from IVF (Committee to Consider the Social, Ethical, and Legal Issues arising from In Vitro Fertilisation and Waller 1983).

11. This recognition of de facto couples was consistent with analogous legislation passed in Victoria, New South Wales, and South Australia and the position taken by the Warnock Committee (Law Reform Division 1985, 18–19).

12. This was National MP Graeme Lee (founder of the Christian Democrats Party in 1994) https://en.wikipedia.org/wiki/Graeme_Lee_%28politician%29 (last accessed September 10, 2017).

13. For further discussion about the role of social workers in ART debates, see Adams (2017, 151–57). Quartly, Swain, and Cuthbert have examined the impact of changes to adoption upon Australian social workers' professional practice in the 1970s and 1980s, including the challenges to the secrecy surrounding adoption led by various activist groups, which resulted in legislative change in the 1980s (2013, 80–86).

14. The Human Rights Act 1993 introduced new grounds of prohibited discrimination on the basis of disability, age, political opinion, employment status, and family status. The existing grounds were sex, marital status, religious belief, ethical belief, color, race, and ethnic and national origin, under the Human Rights Act 1977. See Brookes (2016, 448).

15. "Do-it-yourself" AID (also called "self-insemination"), undertaken at home and outside of the clinic system, was used by an unknown number of lesbian and heterosexual women prior to the 1990s. For discussion, see Adams (2017, 150–51).

16. Speakers included Bill English and Bill Gudgeon.

WORKS CITED

Adair, Vivienne and Chris Rogan. 1998. "Infertility and Parenting: The Story So Far." In *The Family in Aotearoa New Zealand*, edited by Vivienne Adair and Robyn Dixon, 266–70. Auckland: Addison Wesley Longman.

Adams, Jane M. 2017. "Fertility Factors: Infertility, Medicine and the Law in New Zealand, 1950–2004." Unpublished doctoral dissertation, Dunedin: University of Otago.

———. 2016. "The 'Coital Factor': Medico-Legal Approaches Towards Sexual Incapacity and Infertility in Mid-Twentieth Century New Zealand." *New Zealand Journal of History* 50 (1): 88–108.

Batty, Lynne. 2002. "Assisted Reproductive Technology: The Aotearoa/New Zealand Policy Context." Unpublished MA thesis, Christchurch: University of Canterbury.

British Medical Journal. 1960. "Human Artificial Insemination: Feversham Committee's Report." (July 30).

Brickell, Chris. 2009. "Sexuality, Morality and Society." In *The New Oxford History of New Zealand,* edited by Giselle Byrnes, 465–87. South Melbourne: Oxford University Press.

Brinkman, G. L., G. P. Fitzgerald, D. P. L. Green, D. G. Jones, P. Marshall, P. D. G. Skegg, and G. Taylor. 1985. "Issues Arising from In Vitro Fertilisation, Artificial Insemination by Donor and Related Problems in Biotechnology." *New Zealand Medical Journal* 98 (79): 396–98.

Brookes, Barbara. 2016. *A History of New Zealand Women.* Wellington: Bridget Williams Books Ltd.

Bryder, Linda. 2014. *The Rise and Fall of National Women's Hospital: A History.* Auckland: Auckland University Press.

Carlyon, Jenny and Diana Morrow. 2013. *Changing Times: New Zealand since 1945.* Auckland: Auckland University Press.

Committee of Inquiry into Human Fertilisation and Embryology and M. Warnock. 1984. *Report of the Committee of Inquiry into Human Fertilisation and Embryology*. London: HMSO.

Committee to Consider the Social, Ethical, and Legal Issues arising from In Vitro Fertilisation and P. L. Waller. 1983. *Report On Donor Gametes in IVF*. Melbourne: Government Printer.

"Controlled Artificial Insemination." 1978. *Otago Daily Times*, July 13, 16.

Cox, Lloyd W. 1991. "The Development of Infertility Treatment in Australia." *Australia New Zealand Journal of Obstetrics and Gynaecology* 31 (3): 254–59.

Dalley, Bronwyn. 1998. *Family Matters: Child Welfare in Twentieth-Century New Zealand.* Auckland: Auckland University Press in association with the Historical Branch, Department of Internal Affairs.

Dalton, Clive and Claire Rumble. 1985. *50 Years of Artificial Insemination and Herd Improvement in New Zealand.* Hamilton: Auckland Livestock Improvement Association.

Daniels, Ken. 1987. "Semen Donors in New Zealand: Their Characteristics and Attitudes." *Clinical Reproduction and Fertility* 5: 177–90.

———. 2004. "New Zealand: From Secrecy and Shame to Openness and Acceptance." In *Third Party Assisted Conception Across Cultures*, edited by Eric Blyth and Ruth Landau, 148–67. London: Jessica Kingsley.

Daniels, Ken and Gillian M. Lewis. 1996. "Openness of Information in the Use of Donor Gametes: Developments in New Zealand." *Journal of Reproductive and Infant Psychology* 14 (1): 57–68.

Davis, Gayle. 2013. "Test Tubes and Turpitude: Medical Responses to the Infertile Patient in Mid-Twentieth Century Scotland." In *Western Maternity and Medicine, 1880–1990*, edited by Linda Bryder and Janet Greenlees, 113–28. London: Pickering and Chatto.

Else, Anne. 1991. *A Question of Adoption: Closed Stranger Adoption in New Zealand, 1944–1974.* Wellington: Bridget Williams Books.

Glover, Marewa. 2007. "'Your Child is Our Whakapapa': Māori Considerations of Assisted Reproduction and Human Relatedness." *Sites: A Journal of Social Anthropology and Cultural Studies* 4 (2): 117–36.

Government of New Zealand. 1996–2004. *New Zealand Parliamentary Debates.*

Graham, F. M., P. Binkerd, J. T. France, and J. Clark. 1985. "The Development of a Programme for *In Vitro* Fertilisation." *New Zealand Medical Journal* 98 (775): 177–181.

Henaghan, Mark. 2007. "Legally Defining the Family." In *Family Law Policy in New Zealand*, 3rd ed., edited by Mark Henaghan and Bill Atkin, 1–46. Wellington: LexisNexis.

Henaghan, Mark, Ken Daniels, and John Caldwell. 2007. "Family Law Policy and Assisted Reproduction." In *Family Law Policy in New Zealand*, 3rd ed., edited by Mark Henaghan and W. R. Atkin, 223–68. Wellington: LexisNexis.

Hill, Arthur M. 1970. "Experiences with Artificial Insemination." *Australia New Zealand Journal of Obstetrics and Gynaecology* 10: 112–14.

Kampf, Antje. 2014. "Disciplining Male Bodies: Infertility and Medicine in Germany in the Decades after the Second World War." In *Bodily Subjects: Essays on Gender and Health, 1800–2000*, edited by Tracy Penny Light, Barbara Brookes, and Wendy Mitchinson, 157–77. Montreal: McGill-Queens University Press.

Kannegiesser, H. J. 1988. *Conception in the Test Tube: The IVF Story: How Australia Leads the World.* South Melbourne: Macmillan.

Law Reform Division, Department of Justice. 1985. *New Birth Technologies: An Issues Paper on AID, IVF and Surrogate Motherhood.* Wellington: Law Reform Division, Department of Justice.

Leeton, John. 2013. *Test Tube Revolution: The Early History of IVF*. Clayton, Victoria: Monash University Publishing.

McLay, Hon J. K. 1984. "Bio-ethical Problems: The Role of the Legislature." In *New Zealand Law Conference: New Zealand Law Society Triennial Conference, Rotorua 1984*, 50–56. Wellington: New Zealand Law Society.

Marsh, Margaret S. and Wanda Ronner. 1996. *The Empty Cradle: Infertility in America from Colonial Times to the Present*. Baltimore: Johns Hopkins University Press.

May, Elaine Tyler. 1997. *Barren in the Promised Land: Childless Americans and the Pursuit of Happiness*. Cambridge, MA: Harvard University Press.

Mead, Hirini Moko. 2003. *Tikanga Māori: Living by Māori Values*. Wellington: Huia Publishers.

Mears, Eleanor. 1950. "Human Fertility: Some Modern Aspects of Sub-fertility and Contraception." *New Zealand Medical Journal* 449 (272): 384–93.

Mein Smith, Philippa. 2012. *A Concise History of New Zealand*, 2nd ed. Cambridge: Cambridge University Press.

Metge, Joan and Jacinta Ruru. 2007. "Kua tutū te puēhu kia mau: Māori Aspirations and Family Law Policy." In *Family Law Policy in New Zealand*, 3rd ed., edited by Mark Henaghan and Bill Atkin, 47–80. Wellington: LexisNexis.

Ministerial Committee on Assisted Reproductive Technologies. 1994. *Assisted Human Reproduction: Navigating Our Future*. Wellington: Tribunals Division, Department of Justice.

Mitchinson, Wendy L. 1993. "Infertility: Historical Overviews of Medical Perceptions in Canada, 1850–1950', 1–59." Report commissioned by the Royal Commission on New Reproductive Technologies 1991. In *The Prevalence of Infertility in Canada: Research Studies of the Royal Commission on New Reproductive Technologies*, 6. Ottawa: Minister of Supply and Services.

National Bioethics Consultative Committee and Australian Health Ministers' Conference. 1991. *Access to Reproductive Technology: Final Report for the Australian Health Ministers' Conference*. Adelaide: The Committee.

New Zealand Truth. 1984. "Artificial Birth—it's Premature!." June 19.

Northey, J. F. 1958. "Artificial Insemination: A Legal View." *New Zealand Medical Journal* 57 (322): 531–34.

O'Neill, James. 1983. *Alternatives to Adoption: Social and Legal Implications of Alternative Reproductive Modes*. Hamilton: University of Waikato, Department of Sociology.

Pfeffer, Naomi. 1993. *The Stork and the Syringe: A Political History of Reproductive Medicine*. Cambridge, MA: Polity Press.

Press. 1945. "Experiments in Insemination." April 10, 4.

Press. 1983. "Birth a 'First': Twins Due." April 13, 1.

Pool, Ian, Arunachalam Dharmalingam, and Janet Sceats. 2007. *The New Zealand Family from 1840*. Auckland: Auckland University Press.

Quartly, Marian, Shurlee Swain, and Denise Cuthbert. 2013. *The Market in Babies: Stories of Australian Adoption*. Clayton, Victoria: Monash University Publishing.

Ray, Pauline. 1983. "When Babies are Inconceivable." *NZ Listener*, June 25, 1983, 20–21.

"Recommendation 2(a). Human Artificial Insemination: Feversham Committee's Report." 1960. *British Medical Journal* (July 30).

Reynolds, Paul. 2012. "Tāne Māori, Fertility and Infertility." In *The Gift of Children: Māori and Infertility*, edited by Paul Reynolds and Cherryl Smith, 235–315. Auckland: Huia Publishers.

Richards, Martin. 2008. "Artificial Insemination and Eugenics: Celibate Motherhood, Eutelegenesis and Germinal Choice." *Studies in History and Philosophy of Biological and Biomedical Sciences* 39: 211–21.

Smith, Cherryl. 2012. "Tamaiti Whāngai and Fertility." In *The Gift of Children: Māori and Infertility*, edited by Paul Reynolds and Cherryl Smith, 142–202. Auckland: Huia Publishers.

Watkin, Tim. "The X and Y Files'." *Listener*, January 31, 1998, 18.

Chapter 4

An Examination of "Just in Case" Arguments as they are Applied to Fertility Preservation for Transgender People

Damien W. Riggs

In the past, the desire to access gender affirming hormones and surgeries on the part of transgender people required forfeiting a desire to have children (De Sutter et al. 2002).[1] In some jurisdictions this was legally prescribed, with sterilization being a necessary precondition for legal change of gender (Nixon 2013; Wierckx et al. 2012). Furthermore, in the past many transgender people who had children prior to gender transitioning were denied access to their children by family courts in custody disputes (Green 2006). Such decisions often rested on the presumption that staying in contact with a parent who has transitioned was damaging for children (Carter 2006). Early research by Green (1978, 1998), however, challenged the view that transgender people could not competently parent post-transition, and subsequent research has demonstrated positive outcomes for children of transgender parents (Veldorale-Griffin 2014; White and Ettner 2004, 2007).

These changing attitudes toward transgender people and parenting are reflected in the seventh version of the World Professional Association for Transgender Health's (WPATH) *Standards of Care*, released in 2011. This version of the *Standards of Care* introduced what is now widely agreed to be an important area of focus for clinicians who work with transgender people, namely reproductive health. This new focus on reproductive health in the WPATH *Standards of Care* was unequivocal in its stance on the rights of transgender people, and the attendant clinical responses that are then treated as a corollary of this. My concern in this chapter, however, is with how the move toward recognizing transgender people's reproductive rights in the

Standards of Care operates under the assumption of endorsing fertility preservation "just in case" the person decides to have children in the future, when the case at stake is a genetically related child.

My suggestion that the case at stake is a genetically related child is derived from the *Standards of Care* themselves, which note in the section on reproductive health that many transgender people "want to have children," before noting that hormone therapy or surgery "limits fertility," and that, as such, clinicians "should discuss reproductive options with patients prior to initiation of . . . medical treatments" (50). It seems to me that, read together, these three statements rely on a slippage between "wanting to have a child" and "fertility." This slippage positions transgender people's potential desire to become parents within a pronatalist logic (i.e., one that encourages reproduction), and specifically one where the only form of production or generativity that is valued is that which involves genetic reproduction. This ignores other pathways to parenthood available to transgender people, such as permanent foster care in Australia, adoption in other countries (given low adoption rates in Australia), and a partner carrying a child conceived from donor gametes.

To question the "just in case" logic indicated earlier can lead to being misread as opposing the rights of transgender people to reproductive healthcare. While acknowledging the risk of being misread, as a mental health clinician who works with transgender young people, I nonetheless suggest that it is vital that alongside advocating for the rights of transgender people to access assisted reproductive technologies, we must also advocate for a focus on alternate pathways to parenting. So as to resist a pronatalist logic, our advocacy must also include acknowledging that many transgender people may not want to have children. Within a context where pronatalism is actively promoted (through government policies which provide rebates to adults who bear children), it is important that discussions of parenthood do not default to assumptions of genetic reproduction, or indeed do not default to a presumption that all people should want to become parents.

In the following section I expand upon these concerns through a consideration of the literature on transgender people and reproduction, specifically focused on fertility preservation. I suggest that some of the ambiguities that would seem apparent in the literature with regard to transgender people's decisions about parenthood are at times minimized when a normative relationship between "fertility" and "parenting" is presumed. I then examine two narratives of fertility preservation—one from a media report focused on the experiences of a Canadian transgender man and another from an interview with an Australian transgender man—both of which suggest to me the importance of an approach to clinical practice which emphasizes a focus on complexities in terms of decision-making about reproduction, rather than a singular directive toward fertility preservation at all costs. I conclude the chapter by considering additional factors related to reproductive rights for transgender people which also require attention.

BACKGROUND

A key starting point with regard to the limited body of research on transgender people and reproduction is a study undertaken by De Sutter et al. (2002). This early study explored the attitudes of a sample of transgender women with regards to fertility preservation (specifically sperm storage), with the majority of the women surveyed indicating that "sperm freezing should be offered to all [transgender] women" (n.p.). This finding, it would appear, has since served as the underlying motivation for the emphasis upon fertility preservation in the *Standards of Care*, and in subsequent research. Yet, looking at other findings from the study, we can see ambiguities with regard to the attitudes of the women in the sample.

Specifically, only half of the sample reported a preference for having a child in the future who was genetically related to them. Almost all of the sample reported that infertility arising from hormones or surgery was not a reason to delay gender transition. Only half of the sample indicated that they would have frozen sperm had this option been available to them, though younger women were more likely to indicate that they would have done so than older women (some of whom already had children). Finally, a third of the women indicated that storing sperm and using it to conceive a child would be psychologically distressing (given the normative association between sperm and masculinity).

To me, the additional findings that sit around the "core" finding with regard to the importance of offering fertility preservation paint a picture of considerable ambiguity. This suggests that a drive toward genetic relatedness may not be a central concern for many transgender women; that for some women this may be about distress arising from the requirements of sperm freezing (i.e., masturbating in order to provide a sperm sample); and that for many transgender women gender transitioning is a higher order life goal than having genetically related children. In a survey undertaken by myself and colleagues (Riggs, Power, and von Doussa 2016), we similarly found that only a very small number of the transgender or gender-diverse people we surveyed hoped to have children to whom they were genetically related in the future, with those who hoped to have children (a minority) instead indicating that donor materials would be used or that a child would be fostered or adopted.

In addition to the relative lack of interest reported by participants in these studies with regard to having genetically related children in the future, previous research also indicates a number of problems associated with fertility preservation as faced by transgender people. These include some transgender people finding discussions of reproductive organs and genetic materials normatively associated with their assigned sex to be distressing, and the emotional and physical costs for transgender men of undertaking ovarian hyperstimulation and egg retrieval (Armuand et al. 2017; Jones et al. 2016; Mitu 2016).

An additional concern indicated in the literature is with regard to transgender adolescents. At present, the retrieval and storage of testicular or ovarian tissue are possible, though the use of such tissue to produce gametes is only in the trial stages with nonhuman animals. As such, and as Johnson and Finlayson (2016) emphasize, parents must make decisions on behalf of their children about potential future reproductive desires. As I noted above, this "just in case" approach assumes that the corollary of a desire for children is a desire for genetically related children, thus situating young transgender people within a pronatalist logic well before they might otherwise have considered how or whether they wish to have children (see also Fyler et al. 2014).

This way of situating young transgender people is evident in a recent paper by Nahata et al. (2017), who report on a retrospective case review of seventy-three young transgender people who had attended one US pediatric endocrine unit. Nahata et al. found that of the seventy-three young people, only two had undergone fertility preservation; 45 percent indicated that if they had children in the future they would foster or adopt; and 21 percent said they never wanted children. In their conclusion, Nahata et al. bemoan the low rates of fertility preservation in their sample, suggesting that mental health impairments and/or age might have prevented the young people from fully understanding their decisions, in a sense implying that young people might regret not choosing the "just in case" option.

To be clear, once again, my point is not that transgender people should not have the right to fertility preservation. Clearly it is the case that some transgender people desire to have children, and for whatever reasons (as is true for any group), some desire children to whom they are genetically related. Nonetheless my concern is that the recommendation of *fertility preservation* counseling contained in the WPATH *Standards of Care* is based on one specific finding that is not necessarily indicative of the desires of all transgender people. Below I consider two narratives that add further weight to the importance of transgender people's reproductive rights and the need to present a balanced view of future pathways to parenthood (including the validity of not having children).

TWO NARRATIVES

The first narrative that I present here is taken from the aforementioned research project that I conducted with colleagues (Riggs, Power, and von Doussa 2016). In the same project we also interviewed people (see von Doussa, Power, and Riggs 2015 for an overview of our method including ethics approval for the interviews). One gay transgender man whom we interviewed—Tom[2]—specifically spoke about regrets related to not having undertaken fertility preservation:

> One thing I do regret about my physical transition is I feel I rushed into having a hysterectomy and oophorectomy [removal of ovaries] operation, without considering the consequences for my ability to have biological children. Looking back, it stands out to me that I didn't have any counseling at all around the implications for biological parenthood or options I could take before having the operation. I think I had always made the assumption that being trans automatically ruled out biological parenthood so when nobody else raised the possibility, I just accepted that my operation was a part of the transition process. However, in the years since, I've become more aware of trans guys being biological parents, not just prior to physical transition. I'm not sure that I would actually do any of these things myself, but I would like to have been aware that there was the option prior to having the operation.

Tom's narrative highlights the dilemmatic nature of many transgender people's accounts of fertility and parenthood in the context of gender transition. On the one hand, Tom rightly notes that he was never offered counseling—a significant oversight on the part of his clinical team. On the other hand, Tom notes that even if he were aware of his options, he might not have taken advantage of them. Being a retrospective account premised upon reproductive infertility, Tom, it would appear, now considers having a genetically related child potentially desirable, precisely because that is now unavailable to him. For me, this highlights that while Tom should clearly have received more adequate counseling, it should not be treated as an a priori assumption that such counseling would have focused solely on fertility preservation as a route to parenthood, nor that it should have presumed that he wanted children at all.

The second narrative comes from an essay written for *Advocate* by Alex Abramovich (2016), a heterosexual transgender academic. Alex's narrative differs from Tom in that he was able to undertake fertility preservation, albeit not until after he had commenced taking testosterone.

> For as long as I can remember, I have wanted children. For most of my life, I thought that I would carry my child, but those feelings changed shortly after I

> came out as a trans man and started taking testosterone. Producing a genetically-related child was still important to me, but I was no longer able to see myself carrying a pregnancy. After discussing all of our options, my wife, Caroline, and I decided that the closest we would ever get to creating another human together would be to fertilize my eggs with donor sperm and to then implant the embryo into Caroline for her to carry the baby. Unfortunately, fertility preservation, or what is more commonly referred to as "egg freezing," was not presented to me as an option prior to starting testosterone. This meant that I would have to wean off of my masculinizing hormones so that my ovaries would be able to ovulate again. As I went off of testosterone and prepared myself for the worst, I had no idea just how difficult this would all be. . . . But as excruciating as all this was, what continued to be the most difficult thing to deal with was the fertility clinic's treatment.

Unlike Tom, Alex was still able to access his own gametes, but like Tom he was not adequately informed about this prior to commencing testosterone, which clearly had negative consequences for him. Also, unlike Tom, Alex was very clear that he had always wanted children who were genetically related to him. This prioritizing of genetic relatedness, however, led Alex and his partner down a path where the retrieval of his gametes was necessary. This brought him considerable hardship, in terms of the emotional effects of both ceasing testosterone and undergoing hyperstimulation, and the often negative responses he received from clinic staff (specifically in terms of misgendering).

Without for a moment wanting to discount Alex's right to self-determination, I can only wonder if this might have been different had Alex been given appropriate counseling prior to commencing testosterone. Might he have decided that using donor sperm and his partner's ovum would be better for him than the process he undertook? Or, might the retrieval of his gametes prior to commencing testosterone have been a less distressing process? Regardless, Alex's narrative is clearly different to Tom's in that Alex was not operating on a "just in case" principle. Nonetheless, to some degree the norm of genetic relatedness did play a key role in his experience, suggesting that counseling in relation to fertility preservation might usefully move beyond solely advising that fertility preservation is possible. Such counseling might also include discussions about alternate routes to parenthood, in addition to the potential emotional and definite financial costs of fertility preservation.

CONCLUSIONS

This was not an easy chapter to write. As a cisgender (i.e., non-transgender) clinician who works with young transgender people, part of my work involves raising questions about possible future parenthood. I do this not just because it is in the *Standards of Care* but because, for me, it constitutes part of informed consent. This was something that, it might be suggested, both Tom and Alex were denied. At the same time, however, as a researcher critical of pronatalist injunctions and the norm of genetic relatedness (Riggs and Bartholomaeus 2016), I would not be acting according to my own ethics if all I advised my clients to do was to undertake fertility preservation "just in case." In my research more broadly, I am particularly interested in how those positioned outside the norm of genetic relatedness (specifically, cisgender gay or lesbian couples) are potentially "pushed" toward ways of becoming parents which repeat the genetic norm, as a way to approximate the norm and thus secure a somewhat safer place within it (Riggs and Due 2017). If so, I entirely empathize with and understand this. My question in this chapter, though, has been whether or not this is the most psychologically affirming response for all people.

From an ethical position, advocating that transgender people seek a place within the norm of genetic reproduction is likely to produce distress for transgender people for whom the costs of fertility preservation are prohibitive. Storage fees—until such time as the individual decides to use or dispose of frozen gametes—are not inconsiderable, and well beyond the means of many transgender people in the context of multiple other expenses. For example, a nonmedically necessary hysterectomy (which is what hysterectomies for transgender men are classed as) can cost up to 10,000 Australian dollars, and require private health insurance. Costs for testosterone are between 80 and 180 Australian dollars every three months. As such, there is a sense in which following the *Standards of Care* in countries where fertility preservation comes with a range of ongoing costs is not necessarily the most ethical approach. This does not mean that it should not be raised, but the question must be what it means to raise someone's hopes, only for them to be then left unfulfilled. In the case of adolescents, as Johnson and Finlayson (2016) note, if parents encourage fertility preservation and then are responsible for the costs, what does this mean once adolescents come of age and are then potentially responsible for the costs? This type of "just in case" scenario may be even more distressing if, for example, the young person is no longer able to afford the storage fees.

As De Roo et al. (2016) note, as with any form of reproduction, assisted reproductive technologies come with no guarantee of success. While we see gametes and embryos stored for longer and longer periods of time, there is no research to indicate that they can be stored indefinitely with successful outcomes upon thawing. Again, then, what are the ethics of adopting a "just in case" approach if the case in point has a low likelihood of being fulfilled? What does this do to prepare transgender people for the possible heartbreak of infertility? Certainly, the argument in favor of fertility preservation is to potentially mitigate such heartbreak, but it is no guarantee against it. An ethical conversation about reproduction, parenthood, and fertility for transgender people, then, must involve the potential failures of assisted reproductive technologies.

Focusing on the potential failures of assisted reproductive technologies is only one part of the story, though. Another equally important part of the story to focus on is the potential desire *not* to have a child. As Nahata et al. (2017) note, research has consistently found less desire for children among transgender people compared to cisgender people. As they note, this may be a product of gender dysphoria, but it may also be a product of not being invested in reproduction. As such, it is one thing to raise the topic of fertility preservation with transgender clients, but it is another thing to impose an investment in reproduction upon transgender clients, even if under a "just in case" logic. Recognizing that *not* desiring to have children is a legitimate desire is thus just as important as facilitating access to fertility preservation if it is desired.

Finally, research by Moody and Smith (2003) suggests that having children can be a protective factor against suicidality for transgender people. Wanting to stay alive for one's children can serve as a buffer against suicidal ideation. Is this how we want to think about children—as tools to militate against transphobia and cisgenderism? Does it warrant imposing a pronatalist logic upon transgender people who may be considering their future parenting options? Moody and Smith's research did not make these points, so it is important not to put words into their mouths. It is important, nonetheless, to be mindful of the slippages between children, fertility, and expectations about both in a context where, for many transgender people, there are often more ambiguities than certainties. If I have learned anything in my clinical work, it is that attempting to combat dysphoria, distress, or discrimination through recourse to certainties about an idealized perfect world or future is most often likely to fail. Rather than a blanket injunction to fertility preservation, then, it would seem better to have honest conversations about the many roads that may lie ahead, and to try and reach a place where an informed decision can be made on the basis of an in-depth conversation about life as a transgender person in its totality, rather than separating reproduction out as one box to tick.

NOTES

1. I begin by acknowledging that I live on the lands of the Kaurna people, and I acknowledge their sovereignty as First Nations people. I would like to thank Sarah Ferber, Nicola Marks, and Vera Mackie for inviting me to attend the workshop for which this chapter was initially developed, and to all of the attendees for their

insightful feedback on an earlier version. Thanks must also go to Henry von Doussa and Jennifer Power for our collaborative project on transgender and gender-diverse people's experiences of, and thoughts about, parenting in Australia.

2. "This is a pseudonym."

REFERENCES

Abromovich, Alex. 2016. "Trans Men Need the Competent Fertility Care I Never Got." *Advocate.* http://www.advocate.com/commentary/2016/3/09/trans-men-need-competent-fertility-care-i-never-got (Last accessed August 16, 2017).

Armuand, Gabriela, Cecilia Dhejne, Jan I. Olofsson, and Kenny A. Rodriguez-Wallberg. 2017. "Transgender Men's Experiences of Fertility Preservation: A Qualitative Study." *Human Reproduction* 32 (2): 383–90.

Carter, Kari J. 2006. "The Best Interest Test and Child Custody: Why Transgender Should not be a Factor in Custody Determinations." *Health Matrix* 16 (1): 209–36.

De Roo, Chloë, Kelly Tilleman, Guy T'Sjoen, and Petra De Sutter. 2016. "Fertility Options in Transgender People." *International Review of Psychiatry* 28 (1): 112–19.

De Sutter, P., K. Kira, A. Verschoor, and A. Hotimsky. 2002. "The Desire to Have Children and the Preservation of Fertility in Transsexual Women: A Survey." *International Journal of Transgenderism* 6 (3): 97–103.

Eyler, A. Evan, Samuel C. Pang, and Anderson Clark. 2014. "LGBT Assisted Reproduction: Current Practice and Future Possibilities." *LGBT Health* 1 (3): 151–56.

Green, Richard. 2006. "Parental Alienation Syndrome and the Transsexual Parent." *International Journal of Transgenderism* 9 (1): 9–13.

———. 1998. "Transsexuals' Children." *International Journal of Transgenderism* 4 (2): n.p.

———. 1978. "Sexual Identity of 37 Children Raised by Homosexual or Transsexual Parents." *American Journal of Psychiatry* 135 (6): 692–97.

Johnson, Emilie K. and Courtney Finlayson. 2016. "Preservation of Fertility Potential for Gender and Sex Diverse Individuals." *Transgender Health* 1 (1): 41–44.

Jones, Celia A., Lawrence Reiter, and Ellen Greenblatt. 2016. "Fertility Preservation in Transgender Patients." *International Journal of Transgenderism* 17 (2): 76–82.

Mitu, Khadija. 2016. "Transgender Reproductive Choice and Fertility Preservation." *AMA Journal of Ethics* 18 (11): 1119–25.

Moody, Chérie and Nathan Grant Smith. 2013. "Suicide Protective Factors Among Trans Adults." *Archives of Sexual Behavior* 42 (5): 739–52.

Nahata, Leena, Amy C. Tishelman, Nicole M. Caltabellotta, and Gwendolyn P. Quinn. 2017. "Low Fertility Preservation Utilization Among Transgender Youth." *Journal of Adolescent Health* 61 (1): 40–44.

Nixon, Laura. 2013. "The Right to (Trans)Parent: A Reproductive Justice Approach to Reproductive Rights, Fertility, and Family-Building Issues Facing Transgender People." *William & Mary Journal of Women and the Law* 20 (1): 73–103.

Riggs, Damien W. and Clare Bartholomaeus. 2016. "The Desire for a Child Amongst a Sample of Heterosexual Australian Couples." *Journal of Infant and Reproductive Psychology* 34 (5): 442–50.

Riggs, Damien W. and Clemence Due. 2017. *A Critical Approach to Surrogacy: Reproductive Desires and Demands.* New York: Routledge.

Riggs, Damien W., Jennifer Power, and Henry von Doussa. 2016. "Parenting and Australian Trans and Gender Diverse People: An Exploratory Survey." *International Journal of Transgenderism* 17 (2): 59–65.

Veldorale-Griffin, Amanda. 2014. "Transgender Parents and their Adult Children's Experiences of Disclosure and Transition." *Journal of GLBT Family Studies* 10 (5): 475–501.

von Doussa, Henry, Jennifer Power, and Damien W. Riggs. 2015. "Imagining Parenthood: The Possibilities and Experiences of Parenthood Among Transgender People." *Culture, Health & Sexuality* 17 (9): 1119–31.

White, Tonja and Randi Ettner. 2004. "Disclosure, Risks, and Protective Factors for Children Whose Parents are Undergoing a Gender Transition." *Journal of Gay & Lesbian Psychotherapy* 8 (1–2): 129–45.

———. 2007. "Adaptation and Adjustment in Children of Transsexual Parents." *European Child & Adolescent Psychiatry* 16 (4): 215–21.

Wierckx, Katrien, Eva Van Caenegem, Guido Pennings, Els Elaut, David Dedecker, Fleur Van de Peer, Steven Weyers, Petra De Sutter, and Guy T'Sjoen. 2012. "Reproductive Wish in Transsexual Men." *Human Reproduction* 27 (2): 483–87.

World Professional Association for Transgender Health. 2011. *Standards of Care for the Health of Transsexual, Transgender, and Gender Nonconforming People.*

Chapter 5

The Queer Multiracial Family

Figuring Race in Donor-Assisted Conception

Jaya Keaney

It is a warm Sydney afternoon in September, and I am sitting across from Stuart[1] at a large wooden table in the corner of his kitchen. The space between us in the cavernous room seems only to grow with each passing minute. Stuart is the white father of two daughters born through surrogacy. I am interviewing him about his two daughters, one of whom, four-year-old Samantha, sits in the next room quietly watching the children's television program *Peppa Pig*. Samantha eerily resembles my younger sister at four, the same cheeky smile and thick black hair. I am shooting question after question at Stuart about how he and his partner chose the Indian ovum provider and surrogate mother they used to conceive Samantha. I have been trying hard to form a question with the word "race," but the word sticks in my throat. How can the word I spend so much of my days thinking and writing about still be the hardest to say?

Just moments earlier, Stuart had offered the perfect opening for a discussion of race while describing his daughter's body—"she knows she has brown skin; she's no fool." And yet still I could not crack the shell of my own discomfort, the protective carapace of the ethnographer. To do something, anything, to move our conversation along, I ask, "does it feel important to create a link to Indian culture?" Stuart smiles the calm smile he maintains throughout our interview. "No," he says, shaking his head. "We made a very conscious decision not to make a fake link. We're Australian." Moments later, he resolves, "we didn't want to force a culture onto them that is not their family's . . . their family unit is the most important to them, I think."

I feel a churning in my stomach as I rustle my papers. His answer lodges itself sharply in my gut. Race interrupts. Scanning blankly for another question, I try to push away the memory of how as a child I would draw my father with the pink Faber-Castell marker, my mother and sister with dark,

dark brown, and my own face in caramel. I described myself as "Australian" then, though that never halted the continued refrain of "where do you come from?" Flicking my eyes to the fridge, on the lookout for children's artworks, I wonder if Samantha draws her dads in the same pink, or if her birth story sits happily in Faber-Castell brown. On the way out, I tell Samantha that I am brown like her, that my mum was born in India, while Stuart smiles approvingly—the fact that I was mixed race had tumbled out of me earlier, somewhere between placation and declaration. Samantha regards me quizzically, clinging to her father's neck and whispering about the sticker she got earlier that day.

Stuart's family presents an emergent kinship form in Australia—the queer multiracial family created through assisted reproductive technologies. In this chapter, I explore how the queer multiracial family and reproductive technologies alter our ideas of kinship, biology, and racialized embodiment. Where past Anglophone literature, public culture, and clinical practice around assisted reproduction have centered the white, heterosexual, middle-class infertile couple, the queer multiracial family is emerging as a powerful emblem of the drastic changes in the landscape of contemporary kinship. This demands our scholarly attention.

Reproductive technologies like third-party provision of gametes and gestational surrogacy are an increasingly common method of family making in the rapidly changing landscape of kinship. This increase has been accompanied by a substantial "gayby boom" in Australia and elsewhere. Many of these families are multiracial, not least because the industries that facilitate their creation are complex transnational assemblages, comprising gestational labor and providers of gametes from a wide array of countries (Knecht, Klotz, and Beck 2012), and increasingly targeting queer parents as a niche market. Their experiences differ from other forms of multiraciality. Unlike my experience of a family formed through unassisted conception, they cannot draw on dominant narratives of mother's and father's racialized origins to describe children's identities—pink and brown make caramel. The grammars of "birth" and "adoptive" cultures often used in transracial adoption are not synonymous with the structures of assisted conception, where the children often have biological links to one parent.

The queer multiracial family hence raises different questions to other mixed heritage kin arrangements. Race and reproduction are organized in ways particular to the technological modes of their creation. I focus specifically on queer families created through third-party gamete conception (TPG conception), with children of a different race to their parents. Although many other kinships may be grouped under the term "queer multiracial family," I center this form because of its emergent nature, and the specific meanings of race generated.[2]

Race has long derived its power through recourse to "natural facts." The modern concept of race, as I grapple with it, was solidified in nineteenth-century colonial projects and the ascendency of scientific racism, which constructed race as a biological type (TallBear 2013, 33). Although prior concepts of race are widely debated, an understanding of race as a natural-biological category which could be manipulated through reproduction gained particular currency during nineteenth-century imperial projects.[3] Race is not an innate biological truth, but rather a technology for dividing populations into "normal" and "abnormal," designations that are then solidified through their presumed proof in biology (McWhorter 2009). Following Omi and Winant (1994, 14–15), we can better understand race not as a static biological truth but as "racial formations," historically specific systems of race that shift over time, impacted by shifts in other social forces, practices, and institutions. I now turn to consider how the technology of conception through third-party-provided gametes, as an important contemporary mode of kinship creation, creates particular versions of race itself, and its significance for queer family life.

FIGURATION

I approach the queer multiracial family as a figuration, an evocative symbol, a kinship form, or a discursive cluster which indexes contemporary cultural forces and imaginaries. Following Haraway's theory I see the queer multiracial family as a material-semiotic nexus with rich imaginative potential. According to Haraway, "figures collect up hopes and fears and show possibilities and dangers. Both imaginary and material, figures root peoples in stories and link them to histories" (2004, 1).

The family I consider here is both a lived family form, as in the lived experiences of my interviewees, and a mobile discursive entity, circulated through a wide array of particular ways of imagining families.

The concept of figuration also allows us to grapple with how the queer multiracial family emerges, and with what consequences. For Castañeda (2002, 3), figurations are "particular categories of existence [that] can also be considered in terms of their uses—what they 'body forth' in turn." Figuration is thus "understood here to incorporate a double force: constitutive effect and generative circulation." That is, figurations both arise out of convergences of diverse things at a particular moment in time and they simultaneously create new imaginaries and webs of sociality and power.

Particular convergences of reproductive technologies, transnational flows, and discourses of intimacy and multiculturalism, among other things, make the queer multiracial family possible today, imbuing it with affective force.

Many of my interviewees mentioned an increase of such families in their communities, and more than one named multiracial families as the dominant queer family type.

Further traces can be found in media reporting. In 2014 white lesbian Jennifer Cramblett caused a media stir in the United States when she sued an Ohio sperm bank for mistakenly inseminating her with sperm from a black donor rather than her nominated white donor. Explosive news stories of gay fathers leaving Thailand and India amid the crises of closing surrogacy industries in 2015 and gay Israeli fathers retrieving their surrogate-born children from Nepal after the 2015 earthquake bring interracial and/or international collisions to center stage in discussions of queer families, fertility industries, and reproductive ethics (see Marks, Mackie, and Ferber in this volume).

The queer multiracial family is a figuration, provoking thought about the tensions of race and kinship in the present reproductive moment. This family "worlds" particular notions of what race is, and how it operates in connection with reproduction and queerness. I center this figure as a way to trace forms of desire, attachment, and kinship across racial lines. They become imaginable through TPG conception. In Haraway's (2004, 1) words, there are "possibilities and dangers" involved in these worldings.

ATHWART ETHNOGRAPHY

My conceptual engagement and in-depth interview method are steeped in a feminist epistemological tradition which grasps knowledge creation as embodied (Skeggs 2001; Haraway 1988). Understanding all knowledge as situated knowledge, formed through the apparatus of particular sensate bodies, involves turning to the particularity of lived experience. In-depth interviewing offers one method for doing this. According to this method, I aim to grasp experience in situated locality, not as access to static, unfiltered "truth," but rather as the result of a specific, context-bound attempt to render culture through individual narratives.

Figurations themselves are narratives, modes of rendering the messy material-semiotic intensities of the social world into figures that offer footholds and routes of circulation. My interview method aims to grasp something of this affective rendering, and the collision of intimate everyday life with abstract forces like racialization and technological innovation. Such structures are made as much in the intimate realm of everyday kinship as on stages of global politics, state violence, and scientific development. I understand family as practice, a *doing* of relations in the grip of the everyday. Ideas of racialized positioning and kinship emerge alongside reproductive technologies in an inseparable double helix, whereby culture and technology are "coproduced" (TallBear 2013, 11).

In this chapter I focus on two interviews which form part of a larger research project. From 2016 to 2017 in two Australian capital cities, I interviewed twenty-seven queer families formed through assisted reproductive technologies. The parents were of varied gender, sexual, and racialized identities. These two interviews, with Stuart, and with Janice and Amy, exemplify a cross-current in the broader research—the queer multiracial family as an emergent form with specific experiences of racialized kinship. The technical and affective choreographies through which Stuart, Janice, and Amy produced their families construct particular processes of racialization, and meanings of race in the family.

Stuart, as implied above, is an Anglo-Celtic man, and he and his Anglo-Celtic partner had two children, each created through an egg from a third party and gestational surrogacy.[4] Their first child, Samantha, was born via an anonymous Indian egg provider and an Indian gestational surrogate, to whom they briefly spoke. When they decided to have a second child, Trish, the Indian surrogacy market was closing, so they used an anonymous Thai egg provider and a Thai gestational surrogate, with whom they remain in contact. They coordinated these multistep arrangements through agencies in each country. Amy and Janice conceived their daughter Mika through an inner city fertility clinic in Australia. Janice is Maltese-Australian, and Amy self-described as white with a Russian grandmother. They selected de-identified sperm from a Peruvian-Australian donor, and Janice contributed her egg as well as gestating.

In crafting a feminist situated ethnographic practice, the embodiment of the researcher is indissoluble from the process of creating knowledge. Just as Janice, Amy, and Stuart's concepts of race are shaped by technical modes of encounter, so too the body of the ethnographer—my body—is a technology for making race in a particular way, through translating my bodily experience of ethnography on to the page. Racialization is both discussed and enacted: we discussed racialized features of children, looked at photographs of gamete providers to spot resemblances, and I fielded questions about my own racialized position. I constantly felt pressure to disclose my racial identity while speaking with many of my mostly white participants, perhaps in the hope of providing some reassurance that I could be trusted with their stories. My writing position as a queer, mixed-race woman, far from dissolving into the authoritative fantasy ethnographer writing from nowhere, proved integral to generating rapport with my participants. It also helped me to find routes through the affective upheaval of difficult material by forming attachments to it, having "skin in the game" in more ways than one.

As I began interviews, the "strategic essentialism" of a shared queer identity that was so enabling in recruiting participants became at some moments untenable, fraying with the interruptive force of race, which foregrounded the differences between us (Spivak 2006 [1998], 205). At times, I experienced this as a vulnerable and injured position generating defensiveness—Stuart's comments seemed to lodge in my body, and I identified with Samantha against him. Yet, I found that such defensive binaristic renderings of racial affinity, understanding the interview space in terms of a clear white/nonwhite binary, also began to fray as I dwelled in the intimate narratives. In their place, more generative lines emerged. In my attention to Samantha's nurturance, Stuart and I are threaded together in a shared commitment—mine in the uncanny recognition of mixed-race girlhood, memories of which structure my bodily experience in the present, and Stuart as an adoring and adored father. Eve Sedgwick's notion of "athwart" guides me here. Derived from the etymological root of queer, athwart is a critical method that, against the defensive debunking mode of much humanities scholarship, emphasizes intimate, sideways movement—not the defensive "against," but the aside of intimate complicity (Sedgwick 1993, xii). This approach attends to openings, lines of intensity and the messy affective potential of "allo-identification," identification with the "Other," which reveals how identifying *as* always already entails identifying *with* (Sedgwick 1990, 59). The concept of athwart guides my engagement with parents' narratives, a method of situated openness that centers the unpredictable and generative capacity of narratives to world different concepts of the intimate life of race.

RACE AS REPRODUCTIVE TECHNOLOGY

I conceptualize race as a technology, which is inherently sutured to other technologies of sex and reproduction. Far from a self-evident quality of bodies, race only comes into being through and with the technical modes we have of detecting it—the orders of things and ways of seeing that form its discursive frame. This is a "somatechnical" approach—the idea that "material corporeality (*soma*) is inextricably conjoined with the techniques and technologies (*technics*) through which bodies are formed and transformed" (Pugliese and Stryker 2009, 1). As numerous scholars of reproductive technologies have demonstrated, "natural facts" are not pre-given, but are formed and remade through dynamic technical assemblages—collections of diverse things that coalesce to act in concert as one entity (Franklin 2013; Strathern 1992; Thompson 2005). Race is produced in the grip of technologies such that it becomes inseparable from them—what race affords is a matter of the assemblages through which it comes into being.

Race is deeply bound to concepts of reproduction. It finds a fundamental site of transmission and discipline in heterosexual sex. This is the literal apparatus of its perpetuation, as newborn bodies are inextricably racialized, and become the site of vast anxieties around the solidity and dissolution of race. Dominant logics of race, sex, and kinship are conjoined here: one's race is presumed to derive from one's parents in a linear biological manner, naturalizing a heteronormative, monoracial family ideal. This is what Weinbaum (2004) calls the "race/reproduction bind." Akin to Foucault's (2008 [1976], 56–60) theorization of sex as a technology which gathers discursive force through purporting to tell the "truth" of the self, the racialized body is presumed to reveal some truth of identity, biology, and family origins. Reproductive technologies, though, disrupt the normative process of sexual reproduction, reconfiguring its terms. In doing so, they reorganize constituent terms of how race, too, is reproduced—generating different ontologies of what race is and does in the family. This is particularly so for the queer multiracial family, doubly ousted from the dominant discourse of family which is seen as heterosexual and monoracial, or at the least, visually intelligible as biologically related.

If race is a technology made through different assemblages, then the conditions of composition are vital for understanding race at any given moment. There is no ontological race outside its context-bound enactment: different contexts generate different systems of race itself. As Coleman (2009) and Chun (2009) each argue, conceiving race as a technology demands that we sidestep discussions over the "naturalness" of race and turn instead to its enactments—the ways it is assembled, comes to gather meaning and enact force in different ways depending on the contexts in which it congeals. We must attend to the specific technological affordances of donor conception if we are to grasp how race is encountered and done in the queer multiracial family.

SELECTING DONORS, SELECTING RACE

Using a donor introduces selection into the transmission of race and, in this, ideas around its meaning and importance come into view. If you want a sperm or egg donor in Australia, you have few options. All gamete donation must be *altruistic*, given without compensation, and this can take place through a "known donor" or de-identified donors via clinics. The second route is common for sperm donation due to the ease of donating, although there is a sperm donor shortage in Australia. Some attribute this to a range of regulations that in some states require the contact details of donors to be placed on central registers for children to access when they turn eighteen.[5] Due to this, many fertility clinics are also increasingly providing access to international cryobanks, for example, the 2017 partnership between Monash IVF and California Cryobank, whereby Australian intending parents can access US gamete providers for a higher access fee (though not explicitly a commercial payment). De-identified egg donation in Australia, which must be altruistic, is rare due to the invasiveness of the procedure. This scarcity has produced a range of minimally regulated transnational commercial markets, through which Australian intending parents can access eggs in exchange for payment, which they are unable to do through egg providers in Australia.

Stuart and Amy and Janice's selection of racially different gamete providers runs counter to the suggestion in much scholarship and clinical practice that "race matching" is the desired norm—that is, choosing a gamete provider that racially resembles the nonbiological parent (Nordqvist 2010, 1133). Szkupinski Quiroga (2007, 150) canvasses three purposes of race matching: creating physical similarity to both parents, mimicking what most easily registers as biological family, and allowing a family to pass as if conceived without a gamete provider. This threefold explanation reveals the heteronormative presumptions structuring dominant understandings of race matching—for Janice, Amy, and Stuart, visible same-sex relationships lay bare the fact that they required assistance to conceive. They contravene the idea that race matching is the norm, thus requiring different analytical tools to make sense of their queer family experiences.

Stuart and Janice and Amy were each given catalogs of potential gamete providers, and the modes of cataloging produced specific possibilities for how they encountered race. In both interviews, my participants asserted race as "unimportant" to their choice. For Janice and Amy, gamete providers were cataloged according to factors like medical history, height, build, hobbies, and numerous race-related designations—including race, nationality, ethnicity, phenotype, and skin/eye/hair color. For them, being asked about race was surprising: "for us it was about the person, the individual regardless of race or background or religion," Janice says. The catalog from Stuart's agency included partially obscured headshots and very brief medical records. They chose Thai and Indian gamete providers on the basis of cost-effectiveness—race was not considered. This framing of racial resemblance as unimportant is wrapped up with technical affordances: third-party gamete conception detaches a child's race from intergenerational "biological" transmission, isolating it as selectable. Here, race becomes both potentially peripheral, as well as hyper-visible—a kinship category to be choreographed.

While pronouncements of race as unimportant might read as incipient antiracist statements, the rhetorics of "choice" that ground the selection of gamete providers can work to mask ongoing racialized inequalities. Cataloging gamete providers by race reinforces the pervasive idea that race is inheritable, reified in genetics and biologically transmissible. Despite decades of antiracist work disproving the genetic basis of race, this popular conception has only gained traction in our current "post-genomic age," where the gene is increasingly the locus of cultural identity and life itself.

Ordering providers of gametes as cataloged options also creates a sense of equivalence, flattening race as one characteristic among many. This is reinforced by the lack of substantial clinical guidelines and critical discussion around race in donor conception industries in Australia. Such is evident in the recent National Health and Medical Research Council *Ethical Guidelines on the Use of Assisted Reproductive Technology*, released in March 2017. The only mention of race is in section 5.1.2:

> Clinics must not accept donations from any donor who wishes to place conditions on the donation that the gametes are for the use only by individuals or couples from particular ethnic or social groups, or not to be used by particular ethnic or social groups. This type of donation ("unknown directed donation") is considered unethical on the basis that it is discriminatory and inequitable. (NHRMC 2017, 41)

In attempting to halt discriminatory practices, this directive quashes actions that may disrupt market flows, and indicates some awareness of the violent racial formations that can be woven into intimate life. Yet it leaves unanswered questions of how to encounter race as a category of consumer selection, and in the future life of a child. The inequality of global racial formations is woven into the fabric of fertility markets, yet race in the selection of gamete providers is overwhelmingly cast as a benign liberal consumer choice (Cooper and Waldby 2014, 64–65; Schurr 2017, 1–2). Stuart's selection of Indian and Thai providers simply because of "cost" is premised on the racialized inequality of transnational bio-economies which are the product of imperial histories that render the vital labor of feminized bodies in the Global South hyper-available and extractable as a resource (Vora 2015). Amy and Janice's experience demonstrates that not all sperm is equal: their clinic said that they could ascend to the top of the waiting list if they accepted Asian or African American providers. They had been surprised, and said it was "interesting" but that it did not ultimately influence their choice. Race "didn't really bother us, we hadn't even thought about it until they said it, it hadn't even crossed our minds."

REORGANIZING THE RACIAL ASSEMBLAGE

The rendering of race as a multifaceted category encountered through catalogs demonstrates how race operates as an assemblage. Encountering race in conception by third-party provision of gametes entails imagining the body of a future child, and how they will engage with the family space. In categorizing available providers, particular primacy is given to phenotype—to a future child's potential physical appearance, with race organized as a spectrum of equivalent embodied options. The visual is a key site of technical production here—race can come into a visceral kind of being through centering an imagined child's body when selecting a provider. Stuart explicitly described selecting their Indian donor on the basis of racialized features.

> She didn't look as Indian as the other options, which is why we chose her . . . she was still quite dark, um but . . . she just didn't have, it's hard to describe, she just didn't have full-on Indian features.

This description presents the extremity of how race is enacted in third-party gamete conception, as a flattened series of features which center phenotypic appearance—visualized here through the technology of photography. Race becomes a set of shifting significations which can be selected and reorganized.

All deployments of race have some foundational relation to visuality (Liu 2017), but in assisted conception by third-party gamete provision the typical constituent terms and chains of signification are rearranged somewhat. Chun (2009, 14–15) describes the visual epistemology of race:

> By linking outside to inside in an effort to make the body transparent, the body becomes a signifier: by creating a gap between what one sees and what one knows, racial markers are placed in an ever-shifting chain of signification.

Appearance is seen to indicate one's racial biology, DNA, parental origins and ancestry, which in turn are presumed to reveal racial and cultural identity. Assisted conception by third-party gamete provision stretches this "chain of signification," isolating and detaching the visual from other dimensions.

This detachment is particularly evident in the way a child's racialized body and cultural identity were separated in my interviews. When I asked Stuart whether he would foster connections to Thai or Indian culture in his daughters, he said it was not a priority, because they are "Australian children . . . they're part of our family." In a different way, Amy and Janice were invested in sharing their own cultural backgrounds with Mika: Malteseness and Russianness are "a part of her heritage and part of her background . . . it's something that I'd like to keep in our family." Conversely, they expressed hesitation about the gamete provider's Peruvian culture: Amy doesn't want to "necessarily over-identify it . . . it's important for her to know who she is and where she comes from but I don't know I'd go so far as to, say, read Peruvian books or stories or culture." This distinction between family culture and racial makeup is significant—it demonstrates the prizing apart of components that are often collapsed in the family space, and distinctions between what is imagined to flow intergenerationally through kin attachment and presence, and what is carried in biology.

Another distinction is the separation of racial phenotype from racial identity. All my participants acknowledged the marked embodiment of their children—"she's no fool, she knows she's brown," Stuart said of Samantha, and Amy and Janice described Mika's "beautiful dark skin" and eye shape. Both of these descriptions were offered in relation to how their daughters are interpellated in public spaces, with strangers often commenting on their appearance—their bodies.

Phenomenological approaches to race in the tradition of Fanon (1986) would position such epidermal hailing, having your skin and appearance interpreted as marked or Other, as crucial in establishing racial difference and identity. These parents, however, leave identity an open question, a matter of future choice for the child. Amy and Janice say, "we don't know how she'll identify," and Stuart, with frustration, describes the race of his daughters as "irrelevant." These experiences separate racial embodiment from any necessary correlation with racial or cultural identity. The body of the provider of gametes is rematerialized in the body of the child, as Mamo (2007, 205, 212) says, but the racial grammars are reframed through transmission. While the provider of gametes is seen to *be* or embody race in a homogenous way, as in "Indian" or "Thai" providers grouped by phenotype, the children "have" race as a quality that they might attach to or deploy given the right circumstances, but not necessarily. This resonates closely with Castañeda's (2002, 92) description of the racial grammars of transnational adoption, where 'insofar as the child has a racial identity (as opposed to racial makeup), the child nevertheless exercises a liberal "choice," such that the child is ultimately self-racializing. Once individualized and detached from a community and shared identity, furthermore, this child can be "loved" as an "other" that is . . . no longer "racially hostile" or "culturally different."' These dynamics may play out in an even more pronounced manner in conception by third-party provision of gametes than adoption because of the family's partial biological link, allowing the gametes provided to be more easily rendered a mute biological "gift."

QUEER LOVE IN POST-RACIAL TIMES

Perhaps the starkest reordering of constituent components of race in conception by third-party provision of gametes is the separation of race from racism. Contrary to a vast critical race literature which locates race *in* the racist event, my participants make a claim to race existing as distinct from its interpellation within a racist system (Fanon 1986; Liu 2017, 134–35). When asked if he had considered the prospect of his children facing racism, Stuart quickly responded "no, not racism"; similarly, Janice and Amy said "not at all . . . racism isn't something that we're sort of too concerned about." Racism is cut away from bodily difference in a rapid, affectively charged way, rendering race as an innate, biological quality that exists independent of oppressive structures of racialization. There was a palpable sense of awkwardness in the air in both interviews when I asked about racism, and I felt myself morphing into Ahmed's (2010, 65–68) killjoy, too wilful, too brown, obstructing easy happiness by refusing to let go of the injury. The reconfigurations of how biology is thought in conception by third-party provision of gametes mean that race can be thought to exist as a form of skin-deep difference in a unified family unit.

Relocating race to the space of liberal "choice" is enabled by the way fertility industries address individuals as autonomous citizen-consumers (Schurr 2016, 1–22). Though it might appear as antiracist potential, this flattening of race operates as a new kind of racism precisely through detaching racism from race. This racism consists in the uprooting of race from heavy histories and unequal geographies, remaking it instead as a sanitized or settled choice, an erasure of the violences of difference within the loving embrace of the family space.

Such renderings of race are produced within the post-racial imaginary of contemporary Australia. For Alana Lentin (2016), the post-racial constructs racism as both "frozen" and "motile"—fixed at an historical "elsewhere" such as colonialism or apartheid, and yet also generalized to apply to virtually any instance involving race, a universalized quality detached from structural conditions of possibility. Racism within this discursive horizon is most comfortably narrated as an "event"—a public utterance that can be ousted onto the body "out there," and managed through the "three D's": "deflection, distancing, and denial" (Lentin 2016, 2). My participants' swift disavowal plays out the deflection of racism as an elsewhere, an affectively dense taint ousted from the queer family home.

Post-racial discourse locates racism outside the intimate sphere, while simultaneously enabling intimate cross-racial attachments. For Robyn Wiegman (2012, 258), the multicultural present sees the emergence of "multiracial desire"—subjectivities that long for attachment across race, in modes that contrast dramatically with white segregationist subjectivities invested in a narrative of white national origins. Although no less structured by unequal race relations, these emergent subjectivities have a very different affective charge and a different concept of the nation. Reproductive technologies actively facilitate the emergence of cross-racial affinities, helping to "forge multicultural kinship relations without the crisis that interracial sex as the narrative of national origin begets" (Wiegman 2012, 257). It is not that my participants eschew or disavow race altogether—rather, conception by third-party gamete provision enables them to express forms of multiracial feeling that detach race from sexualized colonial histories, instead moving intimate domesticity to the center in the multicultural present.

These cross-racial kinship formations, deeply intimate and deeply public, find a particular mode of expression in the queer family. After rejecting concerns of racism, participants in both interviews quickly turned to queerphobia as the primary lens for future difficulty. Stuart talked about equipping his daughters with positive stories about two-dad families. Amy and Janice's refocusing was more immediate: "I think more so about her having two mums . . . racism no, not at all." Racism is unable to be easily held alongside queerphobia, which emerges as the primary paradigm of marginality. This follows the discursive logic of what David Eng (2010) describes as "queer liberalism." For Eng, the emergence of a queer politics predicated on calls for marriage and private family life relies on the idea of racism as a constitutive history, now resolved—in Lentin's (2016) parlance, a "frozen" past—with queer inclusion the new liberal frontier.

At the time of writing, the contexts of queer liberal inclusion that Eng discusses feel very much alive in Australian public culture. On December 8, 2017, the Australian governor general signed the Marriage Amendment (Definitions and Religious Freedoms) Bill 2017 as approved by Parliament, thus bringing same-sex marriage into law. This legislative change was pref aced by a voluntary "postal survey" on gay marriage, in which eligible Australians could tick "yes" or "no" in response to the question, "should the law be changed to allow same-sex couples to marry?" Of those who participated, 61.6 percent responded yes, and although it was a nonbinding survey, many parliamentarians cited the results as an impetus for passing same-sex marriage into law.

The months of the postal vote, mailed out on August 24, 2017, and with results announced on November 15, 2017, were accompanied by a wave of queerphobic violence and at times vicious public debate on the legitimacy of queer lives, where queer families were a primary target. The staging of same-sex marriage as a matter for public opinion polling rather than parliamentary direction is a pertinent reminder that queer family-making in Australia, as elsewhere, is a site of culture wars, structured by fault lines of vulnerability and a lack of guaranteed political support. Such a climate produces a convincing imperative for unified representations of queer identity not fractured by intra-community differences, and forms of fortified storytelling which center queer family love. Yet, this rendering of love can explicitly reproduce modes of queer visibility predicated on white-centric subjectivities and "post-racial" discourses. As gay marriage is rendered the contemporary intimacy struggle par excellence, the complexities, violences, and pleasures of interracial intimacy become unspeakable, fading into a settled past where we are now all "post-racial." This may only be worsened in a post-gay marriage present, in which queer people have been included in the liberal democratic imaginary via the couple form. Discourses of queer visibility as primary and singular serve to associate queerness with love, equality, and imminent acceptance, forming queer homes as spaces of morality and making it difficult to think through the complexities of racialized affect and injury which may also circuit through them.

CROSS-RACIAL FEELING

In grappling with Stuart, Janice, and Amy's narratives, I do not want to reject their experiences of cross-racial feeling. Not only are their choices deeply structured by fertility industries, I am also wary of any straightforward advocacy for race matching. Such a critical thrust would erase the myriad ways I am drawn into their stories in complex lines of identification. It would also risk reinforcing the fantasy of clear categories of biologized race and segregationist kinship, doing away with decades of queer scholarship and activism fiercely rejecting the assumption of biology as the natural basis for sustaining kinship ties. The separation of phenotype, racialized identity, and kinship enacted through conception by third-party gamete provision may open new intimate possibilities for rethinking families through the generative resources of queer kinship, and love as a resource for thinking encounters across race in the frame of antiracist "allo-identification." These possibilities, however, will be severely constrained if mapped only through ontologies of race as visual accessory, and the splitting of racism from queerphobia in how we tell stories about queer reproduction. I present the queer multiracial family figuration in the hope that it might offer imaginative resources for thinking critically about how the concept of race is always delineated, encountered, and rearranged by the reproductive arrangements that produce it.

NOTES

1. All names of participants in this chapter are pseudonyms. The ethical aspects of this study have been approved by the Human Research Ethics Committee of the University of Sydney, under the title "Race and Ethnicity in LGBTIQ Experiences of Third Party Reproduction," protocol number 2016/215. This includes approval to quote de-identified interview material in any publications resulting from the study.

2. Not all queer couples require reproductive technologies to reproduce. Queer couples who might reproduce via unassisted conception include a bisexual cisgender man and heterosexual cisgender woman, transgender and cisgender gay men, and transgender woman and genderqueer person assigned female at birth. (Cisgender refers to someone whose personal sense of identity and gender corresponds to the sex they were assigned at birth. It is the corollary to transgender.)

3. The origins and historical trajectory of the concept of race continue to garner vast multidisciplinary debate today. For an overview of some strands of these debates, see Kim (2004) and Heng (2011).

4. "Anglo-Celtic" refers to white people of English and Celtic descent, and is a common racialized descriptor in Australia due to the history of British colonization and the forced migration of large numbers of Irish people to Australia as convicts.

5. These laws differ from state to state. In Victoria (since 1998), South Australia (2010), and New South Wales (since 2010), central state registers are compulsory and donor information can be freely accessed once a donor-conceived person turns eighteen, provided that they were conceived after the date the registers were introduced. Western Australia also has a register (since 2004), but participation is voluntary on the part of the donor. Queensland, the Northern Territory, Tasmania, and the Australian Capital Territory have no specific donor laws. In these jurisdictions, donor-conceived people may ask for donor contact details from the fertility clinics through which they were conceived, many of which keep their own registers.

WORKS CITED

Ahmed, Sara. 2010. *The Promise of Happiness*. Durham and London: Duke University Press.

Castañeda, Claudia. 2002. *Figurations: Child, Bodies, Worlds*. Durham and London: Duke University Press.

Chun, Wendy. 2009. "Introduction: Race and/as Technology; or, How to Do Things to Race." *Camera Obscura* 24 (1): 7–35.

Coleman, Beth. 2009. "Race as Technology." *Camera Obscura* 24 (1): 177–207.

Cooper, Melinda and Catherine Waldby. 2014. *Clinical Labour: Tissue Donors and Research Subjects in the Global Bioeconomy*. Durham and London: Duke University Press.
Eng, David. 2010. *The Feeling of Kinship: Queer Liberalism and the Racialization of Intimacy*. Durham and London: Duke University Press.
Fanon, Frantz. 1986. *Black Skin, White Masks*. London: Pluto.
Foucault, Michel. 2008 [1976]. *The History of Sexuality Vol. 1*. Harmondsworth: Penguin Books, translated by Robert Hurley.
Franklin, Sarah. 2013. *Biological Relatives: IVF, Stem Cells and the Future of Kinship*. Durham and London: Duke University Press.
Haraway, Donna. 1988. "Situated Knowledges: The Science Question in Feminism and the Privilege of the Partial Perspective." *Feminist Studies* 14 (3): 575–600.
———. 2004. *The Haraway Reader*. New York and London: Routledge.
Heng, Geraldine. 2011. "The Invention of Race in the European Middlen Ages I: Race Studies, Modernity, and the Middle Ages." *Literature Compass* 8 (5): 315–31.
Kim, Claire. 2004. "Unyielding Positions: A Critique of the 'Race' Debate." *Ethnicities* 4 (3): 337–55.
Knecht, Michi, Maren Klotz, and Stefan Beck. 2012. *Reproductive Technologies as Global Form: Ethnographies of Knowledge, Practices, and Transnational Encounters*. Frankfurt and New York: Campus Verlag.
Lentin, Alana. 2016. "Racism in Public or Public Racism: Doing Anti-racism in 'Post-racial' Times." *Ethnic and Racial Studies* 39 (1): 33–48.
Liu, Xin. 2017. "Racialised Visual Encounters." In *What if Culture was Nature All Along?*, edited by Vicki Kirby, 134–152. Edinburgh: Edinburgh University Press.
Mamo, Laura. 2007. *Queering Fertility: Achieving Pregnancy in the Age of Technoscience*. Durham: Duke University Press.
McWhorter, Ladelle. 2009. *Racism and Sexual Oppression in Anglo-America*. Bloomington: Indiana University Press.
National Health and Medical Research Council. 2017. *Ethical Guidelines on the Use of Assisted Reproductive Technology in Clinical Practice and Research*. Canberra: National Health and Medical Research Council.
Nordqvist, Petra. 2010. "Out of Sight, Out of Mind: Family Resemblances in Lesbian Donor Conception." *Sociology* 44 (6): 1128–44.
Omi, Michael and Howard Winant. 1994. *Racial Formation in the United States: From the 1960s to the 1990s*. New York: Routledge.
Pugliese, Joseph and Susan Stryker. 2009. "The Somatechnics of Race and Whiteness." *Social Semiotics* 19 (1): 1–8.
Schurr, Carolin. 2016. "From Biopolitics to Bioeconomies: The ART of (re-)producing White Futures in Mexico's Surrogacy Market." *Environment and Planning D: Society and Space* 35 (2): 241–62.
Sedgwick, Eve Kosofsky. 1990. *Epistemology of the Closet*. Berkeley: University of California Press.
———. 1993. *Tendencies*. Durham: Duke University Press.
Skeggs, Beverly. 2001. "Feminist Ethnography." In *Handbook of Ethnography*, edited by Paul Atkinson, 426–37. London: Sage.

Spivak, Gayatri Chakravorty. 2006 [1998]. *In Other Worlds: Essays in Cultural Politics*. New York: Routledge.
Strathern, Marilyn. 1992. *Reproducing the Future: Essays on Anthropology, Kinship, and the New Reproductive Technologies*. New York: Routledge.
Szkupinski Quiroga, Seline. 2007. "Blood is Thicker than Water: Policing Donor Insemination and the Reproduction of Whiteness." *Hypatia* 22 (2): 143–61.
TallBear, Kimberly. 2013. *Native American DNA: Tribal Belonging and the False Promise of Genetic Science*. Minneapolis, MN: University of Minnesota Press.
Thompson, Charis. 2005. *Making Parents: The Ontological Choreography of Reproductive Technologies*. Cambridge, MA: MIT Press.
Vora, Kalindi. 2015. *Life Support: Biocapital and the New History of Outsourced Labor*. Minneapolis: University of Minnesota Press.
Weinbaum, Alys Eve. 2004. *Wayward Reproductions: Genealogies of Race and Nation in Transatlantic Modern Thought*. Durham: Duke University Press.
Wiegman, Robyn. 2012. *Object Lessons*. Durham: Duke University Press.

Chapter 6

IVF and the "Promise of Happiness"

Robyn Morris

In this chapter I examine three recent Australian women's memoirs on the individual experience of involuntary childlessness and the undergoing of in vitro fertilization (IVF) treatment, which one author defines as "*that procedure for losers who can't manage to impregnate themselves*" (Bates 2007, 15; emphasis in original). What becomes apparent in these narratives is that each author is heavily invested in the socially inculcated ideal of motherhood. As Karen Throsby has argued, "IVF, for all its rhetorical newness, is predicated on deeply entrenched problematic discursive resources and practices around the gendered body, motherhood, and nature" (Throsby 2010, 236). Two of these authors do not "achieve" their dream of motherhood, with each describing a crisis of guilt leading to stress, depression, and a reevaluation of their marriages and life goals. I understand their narratives with reference to Sara Ahmed's work on "the promise of happiness." After the diagnosis of infertility they seek "happiness" in the pursuit of the goal of giving birth to a biological child. This drives these women (and their partners) to repeatedly undertake physically invasive, risky, and costly IVF cycles. Ahmed writes that "happiness involves a specific kind of intentionality, which we can describe as 'end-oriented.'" After all, she continues, "happiness is often described as 'what' we aim for: as a self-evident good, or an end-in-itself" (Ahmed 2007, 124). She also, however, cautions us about this aim, end, or promise, which she defines as "quite distinct from the feeling of happiness itself." Many of the IVF memoirs I have read, including the three analyzed in this chapter, describe in detail the aim for a child via IVF. As Ahmed notes, however, "so much happiness is premised on, and prompted by, the concealment of suffering, the freedom to look away from what compromises one's happiness" (Ahmed 2010, 196). This is pertinent to a reading of each woman's account of her repeated disappointments and dashed hopes during the pursuit of the happiness she and her partner believe a child will bring them.

THE PURSUIT OF HAPPINESS, THE PROMISE OF THE PRICELESS

Terms such as "hope," "trying," "success," and "miracle" are common in media representations of IVF. In 2008, on the 30th anniversary of the birth of Louise Brown, the first "IVF baby," journalist Evonne Barry wrote that "in three decades of test-tube births, there has been pain and disappointment—but plenty of joy" (Barry 2008, 88). Just a decade after the birth of Louise Brown in 1978, Rebecca Albury, writing about the representation of new reproductive technologies in the Australian press, noted that the popular press "significantly shapes popular knowledge and attitudes towards the new technologies" (Albury 1987, 43). Arguably, though, much has changed in the dissemination of knowledge since this claim in 1987. We now have online blogs, online infertility support groups, and online information portals and memoirs about infertility diagnosis, IVF, and other forms of assisted reproduction.

In 1990, Sarah Franklin noted that the popular media was strongly imbricated in the "social construction of infertility" (Franklin 1990, 206). Franklin analyzed newspaper articles in the decade following Louise Brown's birth and observed that there was a dominant trope of "desperateness" in the reporting of infertile couples' stories. Franklin focused upon how this representation "affects the formation of public opinion and debate over reproductive technologies" (Franklin 1990, 204). As Franklin notes, "couples or individuals not desperate to conform, such as those who remain childless voluntarily, those who adopt, lesbian and gay parents, or others who parent children non-traditionally do not fit into the desperate infertile couple story, and are therefore not represented" (Franklin 1990, 206).

Narratives of the desperate infertile couple "directly link the 'desperate' desire for a child with the hope of a medical cure" (Franklin 1990, 206). This hope for a cure and the resultant birth of a live baby is, as noted, what drives couples to undertake repeated IVF cycles. Joanne Jones, in her memoir *When the Bough Breaks,* notes that the discovery that she had blocked fallopian tubes put her and her husband Tim on several years of the "IVF treadmill" (Jones 2011, 151). She describes her infertility diagnosis as going "from having an entrenched belief that one day [I would] have children of [my] own, to joining the ranks of those desperate women who consider pinching someone else's baby" (Jones 2011, xii). Julia Leigh's memoir *Avalanche: A Love Story* is both a narrative of hope, in the pursuit of a child through IVF, and a narrative of crushing despair when Leigh realizes motherhood will never eventuate. The memoir begins with these oscillating emotional states.

> For a great many nights I injected myself with an artificial hormone produced in a line of modified Chinese hamster ovary cells. I did this knowing that no matter how hard I hoped, no matter what I tried, chances were I'd never have a child. (Leigh 2016, 1)

As Ahmed writes,

> Commentators have described a "crisis" in happiness, where crisis is announced through a narrative of disappointment. . . . What organizes the "crisis of happiness" is the belief that happiness should be an effect of following social ideals, almost as if happiness is the reward for a certain loyalty. (Ahmed 2007, 122)

The crisis of happiness explored in each of these memoirs offers an alternative reading of both happiness and unhappiness, especially from the lens of gender and heteronormative values. Ahmed suggests that there is a "kinship between the feminist and other figures, such as the spinster or the lesbian, who likewise embody the risk of disappointment (which is presumed to be the proper affective consequence of the failure to achieve heterosexual happiness)" (Ahmed 2010, 583, note 5).

This repeated pendulum of few highs and extreme lows characterizes all three memoirs as each writer narrates the fight to defy the low chance of success, the drain on finances, or diarized dates for having sex during ovulation resulting in estrangement and exhaustion. These emotions are experienced by the couples themselves and by their friends and families trying to comprehend this pursuit of perceived parental happiness. Julia Leigh's *Avalanche* is a raw account of her marriage breakdown due to the stresses of injecting herself with hormone cocktails, of feeling jealous of her fertile friends' apparent ease in reproducing biologically. All the while she was chasing happiness and hoping, month after month, year after year, that she would finally conceive. In the course of writing *Avalanche,* however, and after six years of failed IVF rounds, Leigh looks to statistics as a way of understanding her continued inability to conceive. At the beginning of treatment at age 38, Leigh believed herself to be "lucky, exceptional, or altogether outside the realm of statistics" (Leigh 2016, 26). She notes, however, that "the real reason I didn't want to know about IVF numbers was that I was desperate" (Leigh 2016, 26). She eventually found an independent report by the National Perinatal and Statistics Unit at the University of New South Wales (2015). The report analyzes data collected from all assisted reproduction clinics in Australia and New Zealand in 2013 and

> shows that of 71,516 treatment cycles only 18.2 percent resulted in a live birth. Regardless of the age of the patient, regardless the exact variant of treatment, most cycles failed . . . It's an industry predicated on failure. The true graph . . . [is] . . . a mountain with one face Hope and the other Despair. (Leigh 2016, 3)

Adding to her despair are media good news stories: "It seemed that every second day a celebrity in her forties was having a baby. I gratefully swallowed the evidence" (Leigh 2016, 23). She was eager to undertake IVF "to fan the flame of hope" (Leigh 2016, 105).

THE IVF LOTTERY

Sheryle de Lacey analyzes the metaphor of the lottery in discourses of infertility, where women are situated as gamblers and categorized as "winners" or "losers" in the quest for a biologically related baby (de Lacey 2002, 43). Indeed, Joanne Jones writes in *When the Bough Breaks* that she is aware "of the *odds* of this most precious of life's *gambles*" (Jones 2011, 25 italics added) and on her fifth cycle says, "this time I am going to win" (Jones 2011, 66). This metaphor of the lottery is also apparent in newspaper accounts of infertility. Jo Chandler reported on mooted changes to Medicare-funded IVF in the May 10, 2005 Budget, noting that it would cap IVF cycles for women under 42 to three a year—and three in total for women over 42. The birth of a son to one couple is described as their "seventh roll of the IVF dice." With "hunger for a child and high incomes" they happily forked out money for "extra drugs, genetic screening, naturopaths, alternative remedies, even pineapple juice (apparently it helps). Anything that might up the odds." They affirmed that "getting a baby was the No 1 priority" (Chandler 2005, 1).

Another newspaper report notes that "Pregnancy is like rolling dice. With Australians waiting longer to have children, fertility experts are helping improve the odds" (Maegraith 2003, C1). In Ahmed's etymological study of the word "happiness" she notes that it has historically been related to contingency in that it is from the Middle English word *hap*, suggesting chances. The word *happy*, she cites, originally meant having "good 'hap' or fortune" (Ahmed 2010, 574). In contrast, contemporary usage, especially prevalent in these memoirs, makes "hap," or "happiness," an objective, a reward for a certain course of action. It does not depend on chance. In these memoirs, in order to be happy, there is a need to plan and work toward the goal of happiness.

It is a drive for Bates, Jones, and Leigh, and therefore the consumption of pineapple juice, having massages or acupuncture, not eating soft cheese, anything perceived to be linked to scientific findings regarding conception is undertaken to heighten odds of happiness. As Karen Throsby observes, however, "an engagement with IVF does not unproblematically constitute 'doing everything possible' because the technology remains one of seemingly endless possibility, always offering the 'maybe next time' promise of success that postpones the end of treatment" (Throsby 2010, 239).

With IVF reward, however, come risks—medically revealed or individually experienced. When discussing the long-term effects of fertility drugs with her doctor, Joanne Jones is told that it could take at least another thirty years (from the late 1980s) for these risks to be revealed. The doctor tells her that "you and all the women on the program are part of that research. Most of the women are willing to take a possible *risk* for the *chance* of having a baby." Jones writes, "There it was. Be a wimp and back out of the program. Be bold and *possibly* be rewarded" (Jones 2011, 17 emphasis original). The treatment of these women as a medical experiment, as a possession or "commodity" of the IVF industry, is implicitly acknowledged in these memoirs. All three describe the effects of drugs on their bodies and minds, of swollen, painful ovaries, of weight gain, poor skin tone, thin hair, of emotional highs and lows. Julia Leigh, after deciding to stop IVF, is affected physically and psychologically.

> I took care not to expose myself to painful situations and made a mental note to avoid grocery shopping at 3:30 pm., which was also school pick-up time when the streets were running with kids. . . . Most of the baby things I collected I gave away . . . my health was a ruin. I was totally worn down, worn out. My skin was bad and so were my hips. It could be just a function of my age but my physiotherapist said she sees a lot of women doing IVF for hip pain. . . . One of my ovaries, about two months after my last egg collection, was uncomfortable and twice the size it was before treatment. There are cysts that weren't there on my initial ultrasound . . . I was worried about some sort of permanent damage . . . I continue to harbour a small fear that in the future I might be unpleasantly surprised by some latent side effect of all the medication and surgeries. (Leigh 2016, 133)

Bates writes that the "whole infertility story is so unfair. . . . And not just for me . . . I'm hearing about women on their fifth, their sixth, their *twelfth* cycle of IVF. Women who have finally conceived and then miscarried. And then started all over again" (Bates 2007, 149). When told by family that she and her husband Christopher are "doing well," she notes, "We're not doing anything. It's all being done *to* us" (Bates 2007, 149). While each author documents in great detail what procedures are "done" to her, any overt critique of the medicalization of their bodies is subsumed by the relentless pursuit of the miracle baby. As Charis Thompson argues,

> reproductive technologies aim to produce miracle babies, and yet they are irreducibly mundane. When they work they make babies and parents. These kind of apparent contradictions are a signature aspect of assisted reproductive technologies. They are intensely technological, and yet they make kinship; they are variously commodified, and yet they promise the priceless. (Thompson 2005, 5)

This promise of the priceless has a very low chance of success. In an article in the *Sydney Morning Herald*, Pip Cummings writes that "If [the Chairman of the IVF Directors Group] were to design a torture for women, IVF would go close to being the worst" (Cummings 2005, 4).

GUILT AND INFERTILITY

When, in tears from the pain of egg harvesting, Vanessa Bates says to her doctor, "sorry I'm such a wuss," he replies, "You're not a wuss . . . I wouldn't go through this for quids" (Bates 2007, 157). So why do women go through this? The authors of these three memoirs all desire to be a mother but they also note that undergoing IVF helped alleviate some guilt regarding infertility. According to Joanne Jones,

> I wanted our baby and believed I'd be successful. As the infertile partner, I felt an underlying guilt that spurred me on to do IVF. . . . Guilt that I was the infertile partner. Guilt that I was somehow responsible for my infertility, Guilt that I wasn't able to give Tim a son for him to kick around a football with. Guilt that I hadn't fulfilled my "role" as a woman. (Jones 2011, 69)

This expression of guilt subscribes to cultural constructions of gender. With so many perceived and compounding issues of failure, it is little wonder that Bates eventually required counseling and medication for depression. For Bates, guilt also comes across as a harsh and again culturally gendered form of self-loathing. She describes her infertility as "failing the human race" (Bates 2007, 14).

Bates's belief that she is failing the human race is reflected in a recent newspaper report by Ginger Gorman on the ethics of the IVF industry titled "In the business of hope: Does IVF offer couples false sense of security?" (Gorman 2016). The report states that after three years of being unable to conceive, a Sydney-based couple undertook IVF. Gorman quotes the couple's initial euphoria. After their first cycle, when an embryo had been successfully implanted, "It seemed astoundingly easy" (Gorman 2016). At the seven-week ultrasound, however, they found that their embryo had no heartbeat. Aileen's gynecologist decided they would "let it [the dead embryo] come away naturally" (Gorman 2016) and so Aileen went back to work. She notes that "I walked around the office for three weeks with a dead embryo inside me" (Gorman 2016). When the miscarriage eventually happened, Aileen ended up in hospital on a morphine drip. She describes it as a "fairly devastating first experience." The article notes that a few weeks later while at work Aileen took a call from her fertility specialist who promptly told her, "By the way, you had a little boy and he had a chromosomal heart defect. That's why you lost him" (Gorman 2016). In a later appointment with the specialist, she tried to explain how hard it had been to unexpectedly be told the sex of her dead baby while sitting at her desk in the middle of an ordinary workday. The specialist, "looked at me quite blankly and said, '[w]e don't like to coddle our women so we tend to just rip the Band-Aid off'" (Gorman 2016).

In addition to the physical toll on their bodies, the emotional highs and lows result in a diagnosis of depression for both Julia Leigh and Joanne Jones. Vanessa Bates's memoir *Legs Up and Laughing* is in many ways a happy-ever-after story for she does achieve the IVF promise of happiness in giving birth to a child. She also, however, describes how the IVF process had her feeling "worthless . . . angry, excluded, weary and generally lost" (Bates 2007, 140). She notes that her husband also feels this way and concludes that her feelings cannot simply be attributed to the drug Lucrin but are part of a "story of aching, emptiness and obsession and sacrifice" (Bates 2007, 161). Early in the memoir she describes the pain of having a catheter inserted into her cervix to pump through dye so that she feels like "crying and vomiting all at once" (Bates 2007, 12). Later that evening a male friend calls her to describe his experience of IVF which he describes as a "humiliation" because he was put in a private room "and told to ejaculate into a jar . . . and hand the jar to a nurse" (Bates 2007, 13). Bates reacts with anger and sarcasm and "feel[s] like punching him in the face" (Bates 2007, 13). When she tries to point out that his wife would have to go through much worse, "he can only partly agree because the 'humiliation' of his experience was so intense" (Bates 2007, 13). Bates continues to use humor throughout her memoir even when she is recounting the pain of a vaginal ultrasound which she names Dildocam, such is the familiarity she eventually has with this invasive procedure. It is here that the three memoirs differ. While Bates recounts with humor, Jones and Leigh's narratives are underpinned by sadness and anguish and, eventually, an unhappy sense of resigning oneself to childlessness.

The title alone, *Legs Up and Laughing*, indicates that Bates's story will have a positive, happy outcome. While *Legs Up and Laughing* and *Avalanche* are quite detailed about the painful and invasive clinical procedures each woman must endure, Joanne Jones's *When the Bough Breaks,* as the title indicates, is introspective and is written as a lament for the fact that she will never have children of her own. Her narrative focuses on the psychological anguish of several years of failed IVF attempts and the toll it takes on her body and her marriage. This was in the early days of IVF when there was only a 12 percent chance of success. Jones glosses over the painful experience of egg harvesting and implantation while giving a poignant account of her family life, her fraught relationship with her mother, and the strength of her marriage. This memoir focuses on how she and her husband Tim respond to her infertility as a couple: "never once in the years that we were actively trying for a baby, or in all the years following, did Tim ever make me feel it was my fault, that I was the infertile partner" (Jones 2011, 5). She notes the stress that undertaking IVF and infertility placed on their marriage.

> Statistically, many couples don't make it though. Your health, well-being, finances, and emotions can take very heavy battering. Not to mention careers, friendships, social life, plans and a carefree attitude that never quite returns. In short it's hell on everything. (Jones 2011, 16)

Jones also notes that the cycle of hope and optimism are yet another negative social aspect of the IVF process. It is this cycle of hope that unravels the relationship and eventually the marriage of Julia Leigh. Jones notes that

> optimism is one of the key pitfalls of the IVF program. Your optimism and expectations grow with every successful step of the program. They start to climb with results of daily blood tests. Swell as eggs develop in the ovaries. Leap after egg retrieval, and soar when the eggs fertilize and become your own sixteen-cell embryos, ready for transfer to your uterus. And what happens if, after making it that far, the embryos, instead of implanting, die? (Jones 2011, 29)

In these IVF memoirs this is the promise and pain of the pursuit of happiness. As Ahmed suggests,

> Happiness is directed towards certain objects, which function as a means to what is not yet present. If objects provide a "means" for making us happy, then in directing ourselves towards this or that object, we are aiming somewhere else: towards a happiness that is presumed to follow. The temporality of following does matter. Happiness is what would come after. Happiness does not reside in objects, *it is promised through proximity to certain objects.* (Ahmed 2007, 125; emphasis in original)

Bates, Jones, and Leigh all state that they had always thought they would be mothers. Joanne Jones writes that the first time she saw her future husband she desired to reproduce with him. Such expectations, whether social or psychological, are why "happiness provides the emotional setting for disappointment" (Ahmed 2007, 128). Jones understands that repeated attempts at IVF lead to crushing disappointment.

> Many are the times I wished I could have walked away from the IVF program. Wished I'd never started it. Like a friend of mine who, on discovering her infertility, confided, 'Steve and I are too selfish. We'd rather save the money, buy a farm back in England and breed Labradors. Besides, I don't want to put my body through all that.' (Jones 2011, 43)

In all of these memoirs it is the female body and mind that bear the brunt of these repeated cycles of IVF failure. In contrast to her friend who refused to undertake IVF, Joanne Jones writes about another miscarriage:

> For a while the lights went out inside me. I could not see my way past this latest failure. . . . I was empty of emotional, physical, and spiritual energy. Tim was a continuing support. But he didn't grieve each time like I did. He focused on the next task, the next job that demanded his attention. It wasn't his body that had borne the process. It wasn't his mind that had held vigil over the embryos or his psyche that thrashed like a netted fish, seeking a solution, an explanation. *Resolution*. (Jones 2011, 54; emphasis in original)

Each writer repeatedly describes her body as either a failure or a miracle. To their doctors (all male), their body is mechanized: tested for its faults and modified for its inefficiencies. Facing IVF failure, Jones and Leigh undertake a reassessment of their life goals, expectations and sense of self. Maggie Kirkman's work has long examined how women who are infertile deal with the trauma of having to construct revised life narratives in which biological motherhood is not an option. Kirkman suggests that narratives of infertility are "embedded in their cultures. They can be seen to convey expectations of how such narratives should be constructed and how the lives they reflect should be lived" (Kirkman 2002, 61). Kirkman's findings are based on oral interviews with thirty-one volunteers who described themselves as infertile. She argues that for women who envisaged themselves as a mother, to find they were infertile was a disruptive "unexpected event which somehow had to be accommodated within the existing plot of life, or provoke a revision of the plot" (Kirkman 2002, 61).

For Jones and Leigh, the writing of their IVF journey as both failure and as a new life-path requires deep fortitude, enabling each author to look back while also looking forward to a revised definition of happiness. This revision, though, is still linked to failure, to gender, and to a heteronormative social script. It is a resignation of wretchedness and not an embracing of alternative models of happiness. As Ahmed suggests, "unhappiness is not our end point. If anything, the experience of being outside the very ideals that are presumed to enable a good life still gets us something. It is the resources we develop in sharing such experiences that might form the basis of alternative models of happiness" (Ahmed 2007, 135).

Indeed, this notion of "alternative models of happiness" is a distinct feature of each of Jones and Leigh's memoirs. As Ahmed suggests in "Killing Joy," in refusing to be constrained by pursing the ideal of happiness, individuals can pursue other options and other life paths (Ahmed 2010, 593). Indeed, the crisis of sorrow experienced by these writers might offer us "a different angle on happiness, not because it teaches us what it is like or must be like to be a stranger but because it might estrange us from the very happiness of the familiar" (Ahmed 2010, 573). At 40 years of age, Jones is diagnosed with clinical depression after eight rounds of IVF treatments and several miscarriages. What she turns to, as a new model of happiness, is the joy her pet therapy Labrador Dougal brings to seriously ill people in hospital. Post-IVF, Julia Leigh notes a similar shift in focus.

> What I try to hold onto—now that the treatment has failed—is a commitment to love widely and intensely. *Tenderly.* In ways I would not have previously expected . . . To unshackle my love from the great love I wanted to give my own child. (Leigh 2016, 133)

In this sense, perhaps these IVF memoirs could indeed offer what Ahmed refers to as "an alternative social promise" (Ahmed 2007, 135) regarding definitions of what it might mean to be happy or unhappy.

WORKS CITED

Ahmed, Sara. 2007. "Multiculturalism and the Promise of Happiness." *New Formations* 63 (Winter): 121–37.

———. 2010. *The Promise of Happiness*. Durham: Duke University Press.

———. 2010. "Killing Joy: Feminism and the History of Happiness." *Signs: Journal of Women in Culture and Society* 35 (3): 71–93.

Albury, Rebecca. 1987. "Babies on Ice: Aspects of the Australian Press Coverage of IVF." *Australian Feminist Studies* 4 (Autumn): 43–71.

Barry, Yvonne. 2008. "IVF: 30 Years of Giving Life." *Sunday Herald Sun*, July 30.

Bates, Vanessa. 2007. *Legs Up and Laughing*. Sydney: Murdoch Books.

Chandler, Jo. 2005. "The Politics of IVF." *Insight, The Age*, April 3.

Cummings, Pip. 2005. "The IVF Roller-Coaster." Health and Science, *The Sydney Morning Herald*, June 30.

de Lacy, Cheryl. 2002. "IVF as Lottery or Investment: Contesting Metaphors in Discourses of Infertility." *Nursing Inquiry* 9 (1): 43–51.

Franklin, Sarah. 1990. "Deconstructing 'Desperateness': The Social Construction of Infertility in Popular Media Representations." In *The New Reproductive Technologies*, edited by Maureen McNeil, Ian Varcoe, and Steven Yearley, 200–29. London: Macmillan.

Gorman, Ginger. 2016. "In the Business of Hope: Does IVF Offer Couples False Sense of Security?" *Newscom*, January 23, 2016. http://www.news.com.au/lifestyle/parenting/pregnancy/in-the-business-of-hope-does-ivf-offer-couples-false-sense-of-security/news-story/258d7b81a249c9440c80c98581087566 (Last accessed February 2, 2017).

Jones, Joanne. 2011. *When the Bough Breaks.* Sydney: Finch Publishing.

Kirkman, Maggie. 2002. "Moving on, Living in the Subjunctive Mode: Revising Autobiographical Narratives after Infertility." In *The Fertile Imagination: Narratives of Reproduction,* edited by Maggie Kirkman, JaneMaree Maher, and Kay Torney Souter, 59–82. Bundoora: Meridian.

Leigh, Julia. 2016. *Avalanche: A Love Story.* Harmondsworth: Penguin.

Maegraith, Donna. 2013. "Misconception." Feature. *The Australian,* November 22, 2003, C1.

National Perinatal and Statistics Units Report, University of New South Wales. 2015. *Assisted Reproduction in Australia and New Zealand.* Sydney: University of New South Wales. https://npesu.unsw.edu.au/data-collection/australian-new-zealand-assisted-reproduction-database-anzard (Last accessed November 27, 2017).

Thompson, Charis. 2005. *Making Parents: The Ontological Choreography of Reproductive Technologies.* Cambridge, MA: MIT Press.

Throsby, Karen. 2010. *Governing the Female Body.* Albany: SUNY Press.

Chapter 7

Private International Law and Cross-border Surrogacy

The Role of Analogy

Sonja van Wichelen

Following a significant increase in cross-border surrogacy arrangements and prominent cases in which children were abandoned or rendered stateless, judges and politicians in affected nation-states have called for global regulation (Dearle 2015). The appropriate legal institution assigned to do this work is the Hague Conference on Private Law (HCCH). As an institution which produces multilateral instruments in the field of international private law, the Hague Conference sets out to restructure and streamline legal incompatibilities across nation-states—also known in legal theory as "conflict of law." In contrast to public international law, embodied by the United Nations and its human rights regime, the HCCH's field of operation pertains to private life, ranging from financial arrangements to child abduction and adoption. From 2010 until the present, its permanent bureau based in The Hague has performed preliminary investigations with their member states to ascertain to what extent a Hague Convention on International Surrogacy Arrangements (ISAs) is desirable and feasible. To date, six documents have been released, which include reports on expert meetings, preliminary notes, and background notes.[1] The last report indicates that there are no clear signs yet that a convention is in sight and that further research is needed before the Permanent Bureau deems such an instrument viable and applicable.

In this chapter I examine these documents, focusing on how legal and regulatory reasoning around surrogacy contribute to kinship thinking. Many of the arguments around surrogacy invoke an analogy with adoption. I look closely at how these analogies are drawn and how they are resisted. I examine how these relations draw on ideas of nature, technology, and society.

As a legal technology of reproduction, adoption represents the legal cutting off from kin in one place and the legal "kinning" (Howell 2006) of a child to new parents in another place.[2] No biological manipulation is involved. One can, however, speak of a legal manipulation, one that allows a child to be made adoptable and available for people desiring a child. Gestational surrogacy, in contrast, implies the centrality of biotechnology in manipulating reproduction. As we shall see below, however, the recognition of parentage depends on existing family laws in the relevant country. While it is possible to produce a nongenetically related child through gestational surrogacy (through third-party ovum, third-party sperm, and a gestational surrogate), which brings it into line with adoption, the majority of cross-border surrogacy arrangements take place with the intention of producing a biogenetic relationship between the child and one or both of the intended parents.

To complicate the analogy between adoption and surrogacy, I examine a case on cross-border surrogacy recently concluded in the European Court of Human Rights: the *Paradiso and Campanelli v. Italy* case. Here, the biogenetic relationship is missing and new gaps arise in the conceptualization of legal parenthood. In my analysis I draw from the work of Marilyn Strathern (1992, 1996), Sarah Franklin (2003, 2014), Charis Thompson (2005), and other theorists in New Kinship Studies. The field of New Kinship Studies, which can be said to arrive with the emergence of reproductive technologies, examines the ramifications of scientific and technological developments for the meaning and practice of kinship. My focus on surrogacy's relation with adoption in the legal field is predicated on my interest in what this analogy is doing to kinship thinking and kinship knowledge as well as legal thinking and legal knowledge. I am interested in the connections and disconnections that the comparison with adoption brings to the discussion of surrogacy. I demonstrate that, although the dichotomies between nature and culture, or biology and sociality, are held in place when defining what adoption and surrogacy entail, the subsequent outcomes of adoption and surrogacy arrangements generate biolegal configurations of kinning, of making one's own. Biolegality is that which is produced by law's active reconfiguration of biological knowledge. Biolegal forms of kinned life, therefore, share a common constitution, one that is as much defined by biotechnology as by law.

PRIVATE INTERNATIONAL LAW AND THE HAGUE CONVENTIONS

Private international law is a system of law established to harmonize and determine so-called conflict of law situations where private and non-state disputes cross jurisdictions. These issues usually pertain to marriage, birth, divorce, property, or commercial disputes. The Hague Conference on Private International Law (HCCH) is one of the world's leading organizations for cross-border cooperation and commercial matters. It is an intergovernmental organization responsible for the regulation of private matters across different jurisdictions. Established in 1892, today it includes seventy-five states and the European Union.[3] Over the years it has adopted numerous conventions which aim to harmonize conflict of law situations. The status of children has been a primary focus. Conventions in this area include those on child abduction, maintenance obligations, intercountry adoption, and now potentially international surrogacy arrangements.

Since 2010, the Permanent Bureau of the HCCH has engaged in investigations to tackle the issue of cross-border surrogacy. Preliminary documents have been drawn up which describe the information gathered from HCCH member states and the consultations performed with experts and practitioners in the field of surrogacy. In 2016 an expert meeting was held with a mix of experts from twenty-one states, including so-called receiving states and states of origin in relation to international surrogacy arrangements (ISAs). Experts included judges, governmental officials from justice or health departments, legal scholars, and bioethicists.

The issues identified from the investigations and consultations of the Permanent Bureau focused on two main concerns. The first concerned the legal status of children and parents as a result of conflict of laws pertaining to the recognition of birth certificates and legal parentage. The core impetus of HCCH's research initiatives are the statelessness of children (children ending up with no citizenship because of current legislation) and what is referred to as "limping" legal parentage (intended parents ending up with no legal recognition of parenthood). The permanent Bureau draws on a number of cases to highlight the point that children born from cross-border surrogacy arrangements, who travel to the country of their intended parents where the state prohibits such arrangements, are left vulnerable in light of their fundamental right to an identity. The cases, then, also illuminate problems with the child's legal status regarding nationality, maintenance (financial support), and inheritance.

Second, it was clear that wider concerns were implicated in the practice of cross-border surrogacy: issues of exploitation, inequality, children's rights, reproductive rights, and health policy. Because they pertain to difficult public policy matters, to reach consensus on these issues will be a major challenge. The scope and nature of the proposed convention will be important in trying to negotiate appropriate processes, standards, and tools in regulating ISAs.

DRAWING OR RESISTING ANALOGIES

One could argue that comparing surrogacy to adoption is like trying to put a square peg in a round hole. Each phenomenon is based on different histories, different technologies, and different networks of people and organizations. There are reasons, however, why judges, courts, lawmakers, and publics either draw the analogy or oppose making such comparisons. What makes the analogy compelling? How do we relate two different phenomena? Below I trace the justifications for drawing and for resisting the analogy. My intention is not to pursue a relationship of cause and effect between adoption and surrogacy. Although there are indications that the dwindling supply of adoptable children in developing countries is both cause and effect of the rise of ART practices including surrogacy, my aim in examining the analogy rather stems from an interest in knowledge production. In particular, I would like to focus here on the shifting boundaries of biological and legal parenthood to understand what these shifts tell us about kinship knowledge as well as legal knowledge. As I will expand on below, reasons for drawing and resisting the analogy bring up these shifts.

The 1993 Hague Convention on Protection of Children and Cooperation in Respect of Intercountry Adoption (hereafter the Hague Adoption Convention) often served as a model in preliminary discussions on surrogacy. Experts who drew the analogy commented on the similar impetus for regulation, namely "limping legalities." This refers to the situation in which the legal status of children and parentage were uncertain because there were no clear regulations governing the practice and no institutions which recognized foreign arrangements such as adoption or surrogacy. At that time it was argued that the establishment of a multilateral convention for cross-border adoption would help resolve the problem of "limping legalities"—just as it is argued for surrogacy today.

Experts debating adoption in the 1990s and experts debating surrogacy in the 2010s, however, also insisted that the reason for "limping legalities" should not be the sole impetus for an international convention. Recognizing that the flow of children was generally directed from poorer countries in the South to the wealthier North, lawmakers acknowledged the potential for exploitation (of birth mothers and gestational mothers) and abuse (such as the sale of children). The language of economics was invoked in discussions of both adoption and surrogacy, implying a structural "supply" of children and surrogates available for adoption or surrogacy in economically developing countries and a structural "demand" for children in economically advanced countries (Van Loon 1990, 39; Baker 2013).[4] Such a dynamic could elicit abuse, such as child buying and child trafficking.

Those who use the analogy seem to suggest that, in the global arena, adoption and surrogacy are dealing with similar obstacles and challenges and therefore it would be appropriate to look at similar tools to safeguard women's and children's rights. Among the safeguards are legal instruments, such as "informed consent," which is a critical tool in making sure that the child is freely released from the gestational surrogate or birth mother. Aligning the "surrogate" with "birth mother," by having them sign consent documents, allows the surrogate mother to have legal rights like birth parents.[5] With the informed consent form, surrogate mothers transfer rights of parentage, and therefore rights of disposition—meaning all legal rights pertaining to inheritance and control—to another party (Strathern 1996). Indeed, the informed consent form prevents them from any commercial exploitation, from selling the child to another party, for instance (Jasanoff 2005).[6]

There has also been strong resistance to drawing too strong an analogy with adoption. Among the submissions to the Permanent Bureau, some advised not to conflate adoption with surrogacy. Lawyers indicated that safeguards should not be as extensive in surrogacy as they are in adoption, for the children born from ISAs often had biogenetic relations with one of the intended parents. Lawyers were wary of too many bureaucratic layers slowing down the process and making it more difficult for intending parent/s (who are often also the genetic parent/s) to reproduce. Moreover, the argument was made that surrogate mothers, in contrast to birth mothers in adoption, had the right to regard this as a service they provided, namely, as reproductive labor performed to fulfill a contract between the surrogate mother and intending parents. In this case, the contract should not be about the transfer of parental rights but about the labor being performed for an appropriate remuneration.[7]

The resistance to drawing too close an analogy with adoption discloses a discussion of legal as opposed to genetic (or biological) kinship. It is assumed that children born from gestational surrogacy arrangements, of which one of the intended parents is the genetic parent (usually the father), should, by genetic design of kinship, belong to the genetic parent. There exists, then, an automatic proprietary relationship between biogenetic relations, meaning that the genetic child naturally belongs to his or her genetic parent. Here, the argument goes that the phenomenon of surrogacy assumes an entirely different intention and constitution of family. Whereas adoption involves the abandonment of children on the one hand and the "kinning" (Howell 2006) of children on the other through legal means, the practice of surrogacy assumes an already-established kin relationship through biological means, often via the genetic relationship between the intended father and the child.[8] This apparently neat distinction between surrogacy and adoption has recently been challenged in court. How can we compare biological and adoptive parenthood in the reproduction of a nongenetically related child?

THE CASE OF *PARADISO AND CAMPANELLI V. ITALY*

This case[9] involved a married Italian couple, Ms. Donatina Paradiso (1967) and Mr. Giovanni Campanelli (1955) who, after numerous failed attempts to conceive (naturally or with the assistance of reproductive technologies), and a failed attempt to adopt (because of adoption restrictions and the shortage of adoptable children in Italy), traveled to Moscow to enter into a surrogacy arrangement with a Russian gestational surrogate brokered by a Russian company called Rosjurconsulting. The arrangement—the conception of an embryo from anonymous sperm and oocyte provision through commercial surrogacy—is illegal in Italy while not illegal in Russia.[10] According to the court's documents, the couple claimed that the intended father had provided the sperm, though this appeared not to be the case after a genetic test was ordered by the courts. A son was born in February 2011 who was named Teodoro Campanelli. The Russian birth certificate, issued a few days later, omitted any reference to the surrogacy arrangement, and the intended parents were registered as the child's parents. Upon return to Italy with their child the local authorities refused to enter the child's birth certificate into their register after hearing from the Italian consulate in Moscow that the paperwork in respect of the child's birth contained false information. The couple was then placed under formal investigation for "altering civil status" (forgery) and for breaching the Adoption Act (they went against an adoption authorization which stipulated that they could not adopt a child as young as the child they brought back to Italy).[11]

It was here that the State Counsel's Office made a formal request to declare the child as abandoned and free for adoption. The couple resisted and requested to formally adopt the child. After it became apparent through a genetic test that the intended parents were not genetically linked to the child, the Youth Court decided to remove the child from the intended parents and to place him in a children's home. After two years with no official identity, the child was placed with foster parents and given a new name and birth certificate. Although investigations of their putative criminal acts were still ongoing and not yet proven, the Italian authorities deemed the case serious enough to order the removal of the child.

The couple brought the case to the European Court of Human Rights[12] and filed an application against the Italian Republic under Article 34 of the Convention for the Protection of Human Rights and Fundamental Freedoms in April 2012.[13] The judgment that followed in January 2015 recognized that there had been an interference with the applicants' private and family life.[14] The judgment articulated that the removal of the child by the national authorities was not justified, for it prevented family life from developing. The child had now, however, established family life with the foster family. Even though the applicants were within their rights, the State was not obliged to return the child to them. The judgment of the Grand Chamber in January 2017, however, deviated significantly. Although recognizing that family life had been interfered with, the Court decided that in this case, the interest of Italy's public policy to prevent illegality and protect order weighed more than the couple's right to private life. The child was to be given a new name and identity, and was now declared adoptable.

The case complicates the analogy between surrogacy and adoption. In what follows I analyze what kinds of shifts in thinking about genetic and adoptive parenthood are generated by this particular case and its outcome.

TURNING SURROGACY INTO ADOPTION

Without going too deeply into the legal details of the *Paradiso and Campanelli v. Italy* case—one that raises many issues besides the one discussed here—I would like to focus on the primacy of adoption in a case that dealt with cross-border surrogacy.

It is the nongenetic relation, and the role of adoption, that makes this case distinctive in comparison to preceding landmark cases on cross-border surrogacy. The cases *Mennesson v. France* and *Labassee v. France*, for instance, were such landmark cases.[15] In these two cases of cross-border gestational surrogacy from the United States to France—with a genetic link between the intended father and child—the judgments in 2014 ruled that by not acknowledging legal parenthood or by not providing the children French citizenship, France had intervened in the private life not necessarily of the parents but of the children.[16] Moreover, as family life was established between the intended parents and the children (the children were thirteen and fourteen at the time of the hearings and had lived with their intended parents since birth), it was decided that it was in the best interest of the child in each case to obtain legal identities and citizenship, and therefore for the court to recognize parenthood.

It is clear that the court in the French cases privileged biogenetic connections in their recognition of parenthood. Although the court did not endorse the "right to family life" with respect to the intending parents, it did acknowledge the intervention in the private lives of the children. Their reasoning was based on a child's identity being linked to biological parenthood, and that it was not in the best interest of the child "to deprive him or her of a legal relationship of this nature" (Mennesson, cit., par. 100). France had refused the parental relationship and this had therefore affected their identity.

As a number of legal scholars have observed and critiqued with regard to the *Mennesson* and *Labassee* cases (see Beaumont and Trimmings 2016), the genetic link between the oocyte providers and the children received little attention during the court proceedings. Does the genetic link between the oocyte provider and the child not have as much weight and meaning as that between the genetic father and the child? Does it not go against the best interest of the child to deprive the child of that form of relatedness?

The lack of genetic connections between the intended parents and the child in the Italian case led to an entirely different situation in domestic law, and eventually, also in the judgment by the ECHR. It was because of the lack of a genetic connection—confirmed by a DNA test during the domestic hearings—that the Youth court had requested to free the child for adoption, for s/he had now formally been abandoned. The nongenetic link, moreover, disallowed the child from being represented by the intended parents. The lack of genetic connection barred them from legally representing the child's interests in a court of law.

What does abandonment, or the loss of relations, mean here? Child abandonment, as we have come to know it in family law, is generally understood as the *willful* withholding of emotional, physical, and financial support of the parent or guardian (Bainham 2003). In the Italian case the intentional parents did not *willfully* withhold such care. On the contrary, they were *intending* to parent the child they had helped to create. The status of intended parents, then, becomes destabilized in situations of nongenetic relations. In fact, the nongenetic component turned a surrogacy case into an adoption case. As there were no biological connections, and as the Russian surrogate mother had formally relinquished the child, the Italian court deemed it appropriate that the Adoption Law was applicable in this case.

It was not entirely inconceivable that the court would recognize the intended parents as a de facto family and honor recognition of parentage on the basis of the applicant's right to private and family life. This was, in fact, the situation for the first judgment from the ECHR. If this earlier judgment had not been overturned by the Grand Chamber—the ultimate court of the European Court of Human Rights—it would have started a precedent for de facto families and, one can argue, would have also introduced a *right* to family life, a positive obligation of the state to honor people's right to procreate rather than the present negative obligation to not interfere in one's private and family life. Such a move would solidify "intentionality" as a legitimate claim to legal parenthood. What is the connection between biological and social parenthood?

MEROGRAPHIC CONNECTIONS AND ANALOGIC RETURNS

In conventional adoption arrangements, the woman who gives birth to the child is the *birth mother* and not a surrogate mother. Nonetheless, in the *Paradiso and Campanelli v. Italy* case, adoption law is being applied to a gestational surrogacy case. Such a deployment—though not uncommon in law—does have consequences as to how we see adoption and how adoption evolves in the age of biotechnology where genetics and reproductive technologies play an increasing role (Van Wichelen 2019). Here, new forms of kinship thinking make their way into legal thinking, and adoptive relations entwine with intentional and de facto relations which have their origins in surrogacy arrangements. One could say that the cases illustrate the stretch of the analogy in which surrogacy and adoption are collapsed or, in a Strathernian manner, are cut into one another. The meaning of one phenomenon (adoption) is attached to another (surrogacy).

Marilyn Strathern describes how kinship knowledge is not formed from knowledge in the domain of either nature, society, or technology. Rather, nature, society, and technology form their own wholes, and have their own logical contexts and dynamics (1992). It is in the spaces where they connect that the truth of kinship comes to being or *ontologizes*, so to say. These are merographic connections: "a habit of thought common to relations made through commodity exchanges whereby a person sees his or her attributes in another person or thing" (Sykes 2005, 183). Here, kinship is "a mix of ingredients" and is used "to secure, as well as flex, connections" (Franklin 2014, 5). Drawing from Strathern's work, Sarah Franklin describes how analogical apparatuses are useful "in the effort to characterize how kinships and identities are both signified through substance and substantialized through signs" (Franklin 2014, 5). Taking it further, Franklin proposes that "merographic connection cannot be understood primarily in terms of the logic of the parts it commingles." Instead, it needs to "be analyzed in terms of the effects engendered by such commingling" (2014, 8). Here, Franklin uses the term *analogic return* to designate how such effects can return to the original object of analogy. With this she means to say that analogies do not only work in one direction (for instance, "just like nature"); they are able to "travel back" (for instance, "just like technology") (Franklin 2014, 6).

Returning to the analogy between surrogacy and adoption, we find an analogic return in the legal reasoning of the *Paradiso and Campanelli v. Italy* case. Here, a double analogy (or paradox) unfolds in thinking the substance of surrogacy (it is just like natural production and nothing like natural production, it is just like adoption and nothing like adoption). The double analogy works in both directions and these directions have been demonstrated by the diverging judgments. In law, drawing from different contexts and phenomena is not new. Judges are continually faced with novel problems of parentage and have to find creative and innovative ways to induce and utilize meaning from current and older legislations and precedents. By definition, legal processes demonstrate merographic connections and utilize analogy to further and stretch legal thinking and knowledge. While the *flexing* of connections takes place during court proceedings, judgments and precedents *secure* connections. Once precedents are made, however, it is hard to undo the finiteness of the judgments which created them.

In sum, biotechnology, assisted reproduction, and the new genetics bring novel problems to legal thinking. Rather than assuming that law lags behind, or that future regulation will restore a previous equilibrium, it is more accurate to adopt the view that an active reorganization of legal and biological knowledge is taking place which displaces—or puts on hold—conventional understandings of kinship. By activating different legal domains with their own knowledge systems, law can contribute to remodeling kinship.[17] In society, such activation comes from our own engagements in who defines and how we define our kin. Biology or nature can intervene but so can technologies, including legal technologies. Such an exchange can—as Franklin notes—produce new classifications of "biological relatives" (2013). Translated to law, we can argue that *biolegal* exchange could similarly produce new forms of "legal relatives."

BIOLEGALITY IN THE GLOBAL REPRODUCTIVE MARKET

The move in many countries toward non-anonymity in domestic policies on assisted reproduction and surrogacy attests to a view that the genetic relationship between the oocyte donor and the child is more important to the child's identity than thought previously. In the language of rights and international law, one can argue that the geneticization of identity translates in the doctrine of "the right to know."[18] Although the debate surrounding anonymity in donor-conceived conceptions remains a highly contentious issue in the field of bioethics, from a human rights perspective the "right to know" has been firmly placed in conventions as well as domestic laws. This is especially noticeable in the adoption field where "open adoption" is gaining traction in Northern American, European, Australian, and Pacific locations and is replacing the practice of secret adoptions (Modell 2002; Howell 2009; Yngvesson 2010; Marks 2017; Adams in this volume).

The rise and prominence of genetics and biotechnology actively reworked this meaning of blood relationships. Couched in the increasing Euro-American interest in genetic origins (Nash 2002, 2004; Rose 2009), adoptees and donor-conceived children increasingly depend conceptually and commercially on the global "kinning" of genetic connectivity. This has to do with the resolutely biologistic construal of DNA as the real substance of kinship itself (Hamilton and Faubion 2007: 550). The geneticization of human identity collapses identity, and by proxy, kinship, with biology and advances a discourse of determinism. This development has strengthened the directive toward openness in the domestic sphere. We can see similar tendencies in the transnational regulation of intercountry adoption as well as the preliminary work for a possible future convention on surrogacy.

When genetics—or biology—is allowed to travel across borders, while social, intentional, or de facto relations cannot, how can we think about regulating the private in the broader context of the social and the global?

The legal scholar Horatia Muir Watt contends that the focus of private international law has always been on enabling capacities, rather than that of disciplining (2011, 427). Private international law, she further argues, is founded on the schism between law and politics, and between the public and the private. It is time, she argues, that private international law matures into an international law instrument where its political function is reappropriated.

> Private international law should reclaim its governance potential and work to fill the holes created either by excluding or denying non-state authority. Paradoxically, when domesticated and thus reduced to dealing with the "private" sphere, it was actually disabled from taking the 'private' seriously. To a large extent, "privatising" international law meant reducing its status—like that of classical private law—to the merely facilitative. Used to enable but not to discipline, it was prevented from identifying and regulating private economic power, which it was complicit in unleashing from public constraints. (2011, 389)

In agreement with this observation, I argue that a future multilateral private law instrument regulating surrogacy would need to make further efforts to ensure that solutions work against, rather than with reproductive markets and bioeconomies (van Wichelen 2017). Put differently, it would need to acknowledge the intricately linked social, political, and global context of private (family) lives. As in adoption, this would mean not only exploring the opportunities, needs, and rights of intending parents (or the limping legalities for their families). More importantly, it would also mean investigating and addressing the inherent global inequalities constitutive of global reproductive markets. While the work on parentage and kinship thinking seems separate from the problem of markets, I would contend that they are mutually constitutive. Without the legal recognition of genetic parenthood, gestational surrogacy would lose its legitimacy. Similarly, without the legal recognition of adoptive parenthood, adoption would lose its validity. In short, genetics and legalities are enabling forces of knowledge. Within a context of reproductive economies, such knowledges are able to *kin* or *de-kin* relations, and to produce legitimate or illegitimate families.

CONCLUSION

Strathern describes how Euro-American kinship ties are defined by merging (or cutting) nature into culture, and the other way around, culture into nature: "biological relatedness—blood ties—can be cut by failure to accord social recognition (someone is forgotten), just as social relationships can be cut by appeal to biological principles (dividing 'real' kin from others)" (1996, 53). Genetic kinship and adoptive kinship appeal to these divisions. Within their own contexts, they have formed or are in the process of forming knowledge about what constitutes (adoptive and genetic) parenthood. Here, different forms of kinship knowledge intersect and are unmoored from their contexts; they not only evoke new substance but also change each other's potential.

In this chapter I have explored these potentialities by examining the changes that knowledge practices around adoption and surrogacy are undergoing in a biotechnological age that sees itself as controlling nature and transgressing borders. The advancement of assisted reproductive technologies reinforced the medicalization of infertility. It also allowed family making to become more attainable. Various forms of parenthood—such as biological, genetic, adoptive, intentional, or de facto parenthood—are therefore firmly entangled in reproductive services and legal technologies should be understood as integral to reproductive technologies.

Certainly, adoption and family-making practices based on reproductive technologies are different phenomena, relying on different histories, legalities, and scientific practices. In this chapter I have demonstrated, however, that contemporary applications of adoption knowledge in law and regulation exist in tandem with new knowledge practices involving reproductive technologies. Moreover, the geneticization of kinship—dominant in public discourse today—affects intentional, de facto, and adoptive families as much as it does biogenetic families. It is to these ends that we cannot separate nature and biology, or society, technology, and culture, from the broader reproductive landscape. Nor can we separate the discussion of kinship thinking from the domains of the reproductive market. The relationship between the life sciences, law, and markets in the globalization of adoption reflects how we legitimate life in late capitalism. With the globalization of reproductive technologies, and new reproductive phenomena like cross-border surrogacy, such legitimation work (whether from society, science, or law) becomes more pressing.

NOTES

1. (1) "Report of the February 2016 meeting of the Experts," (2) "Background Note for the meeting of the Experts," (3) "The Parentage / Surrogacy Project: An updating note (Prel. Doc. No 3 A of February 2015)," (4) "The desirability and feasibility of further work on the Parentage / Surrogacy Project (Prel. Doc. No 3 B of March 2014) and its accompanying 'Study of Legal Parentage and the Issues Arising from International Surrogacy Arrangements' (Prel. Doc. No 3 C of March 2014)," (5) "Preliminary Report on international surrogacy arrangements," and (6) "Preliminary Note on the private international law issues surrounding the status of children." All documents concerning the preliminary investigations on cross-border surrogacy and the feasibility of a Hague Convention on International Surrogacy Arrangements (ISAs) can be found at https://www.hcch.net/en/projects/legislative-projects/parent age-surrogacy.

2. Different jurisdictions deal with adoption in different ways. These pertain to the rules of domestic adoption. International adoption, however, as regulated through the Hague Adoption Convention, primarily concerns full adoptions, meaning that the ties with birthparents are legally cut off.

3. This means that many states are not included, among them most of the countries in Africa, the Middle East, and Southeast Asia.

4. Research has indicated that the vectors of movement are more complex than a simple flow from the Global North to the Global South. Both in adoption and surrogacy there are flows among richer countries. With respect to adoption, countries such as the Netherlands, Sweden, and Israel also adopt from the United States. Similarly, with respect to surrogacy, intending parents from Australia and Japan travel to the United States. Both have to do with the regulatory regimes which facilitate adoption and surrogacy in states like California, New Jersey, and Nevada. Nonetheless, these movements are often costly and are inaccessible for many prospective adopters or intended parents who turn to more affordable options in the Global South (see also Marks, Mackie, and Ferber in this volume).

5. The timing of consent, however, can be different in adoption and surrogacy. In most countries in Europe, relinquishing a child for adoption, and thereby transferring parental rights to the state or to prospective adoptive parents, occurs after birth. In some states in the United States where private adoption is allowed there are mothers who relinquish before the birth of the child. In contrast, in states where commercial surrogacy is allowed (such as California), it is in the surrogacy contract before conception where parental rights are relinquished to intending parents.

6. One could say, then, that the commercial property rights do not belong to the surrogate, but to the intermediaries or agencies brokering and facilitating the surrogacy arrangements: lawyers, medical physicians, social workers, and agents and agencies who all "add labor" to the material (Landecker 1999; Hoeyer and Hogle 2014) and allow informed consent documents to be an integral part of the reproductive economy (Cooper and Waldby 2014; Waldby and Mitchell 2006).

7. This might also be true of some adoption cases where a pregnant woman enters into an agreement with intending parents to relinquish her child as happens in private adoptions in some states in the United States.

8. The majority of cross-border surrogacy cases involve genetic material of an intended father, but there are cases where the gestational surrogate bears a child with genetic material from both intending parents.

9. *Paradiso and Campanelli v. Italy*, Application No. 25358/12. For the full judgment, see: http://hudoc.echr.coe.int/sites/eng/pages/search.aspx?i=001-150770 (last accessed September 30, 2018).

10. According to the proceedings, the couple initially thought that there was a genetic link between the intended father and the child. They claimed that they only found out that the father was not genetically linked when they were obliged to take a genetic test by the court.

11. In the adoption world, every country has its own regulations about age restrictions. These concern the maximum age of prospective adopters and also the maximum age of adoptive children. The rationale behind age restrictions for adopters is to minimize the chance that the child has to deal with premature death or disease of the adoptive parents. The reason for having restrictions on the age of the adoptive child is to promote early adoptions, for research has proven that attachment occurs earlier rather than later in life.

12. The case originated in an application no. 25358/12.

13. The applicants also lodged an application on behalf of the child who, according to the birth certificate issued by the Russian authorities on March 1, 2011, was their son, born on February 27, 2011, and was named Teodoro Campanelli. This application was denied after it became apparent that there was no genetic link between the intended father and child.

14. This is stipulated in article 8 of the European Convention of Human Rights (ECHR).

15. Case of *Mennesson v. France*, Application no. 65192/11, Judgment June 26, 2014, and Case of *Labassee v. France*, Application no. 65941/11, Judgment June 26, 2014. The same judges chaired the two cases.

16. The gestational surrogate in the case of *Mennesson v. France* gave birth to twins in California. The gestational surrogate in the *Labessee v. France* case gave birth to a child in Minnesota.

17. See Franklin (2014) for an account of "activation" in kinship thinking.

18. The principle of "the right to know" is articulated in a number of ways. The Convention on the Rights of the Child (CRC) includes it as "the right to know his or her parents" (Article 7.1), and when this relationship is severed, the state is obliged to provide assistance and protection to reestablish the child's identity (Article 8.2). The CRC also has a clear directive that in educating the child, (adoptive) parents have an important role to socialize the child about the child's own cultural identity, language, values (including national values), and civilizations (Article 29). Nevertheless, the Hague Adoption Convention notes that the identity of the mother and the father may not be disclosed when the laws in the State of Origin respect the privacy of the birth-parents (Article 16). Although Article 30 stipulates that "authorities are to ensure that information held by them concerning the child's origin, in particular information concerning the identity of his or her parents, as well as the medical history, is preserved," and in point 2, that "they shall ensure that the child or his or her representative has

access to such information" this is only applicable "in so far as it is permitted by the law of that State" (30.2). There remains, then, a double standard in the formulations of the right to know, namely that, as it stands, it only applies to children born in states that allow access to adoption records. Nonetheless, although implicit, there is a clear directive in these conventions that openness is the way forward, and that states that continue to have closed records are encouraged and assisted to work toward openness.

WORKS CITED

Bainham, Andrew. 2003. "International Adoption from Romania – Why the Moratorium Should Not Be Ended." *Child and Family Law Quarterly* 15 (2003): 223.

Baker, Hannah. 2013. "A Possible Future Instrument on International Surrogacy Arrangements: Are There 'Lessons' to be Learnt from the 1993 Hague Intercountry Adoption Convention?" *International Surrogacy Arrangements: Legal Regulation at the International Level*, edited by Katarina Trimmings and Paul R. Beaumont, 411–26. Oxford: Hart Publishing.

Beaumont, Paul and Katarina Trimming. 2016. "Recent Jurisprudence of the European Court of Human Rights in the Area of Cross-border Surrogacy: Is there Still a Need for Global Regulation of Surrogacy?" Centre for Private International Law, University of Aberdeen, Working Paper no. 2016/4. https://www.abdn.ac.uk/law/research/working-papers-455.php (Last accessed November 14, 2017).

Cooper, Melinda and Catherine Waldby. 2014. *Clinical Labor: Tissue Donors and Research Subjects in the Global Bioeconomy*. Durham: Duke University Press.

Council of Europe, Right to Respect for One's Private and Family Life, His Home and His Correspondence, European Convention on Human Rights (ECHR), Art 8.

Dearle, Marcus. 2015. "Time for International Surrogacy Regulation: The Complex Minefield of Global Surrogacy Law is Catching People Out and the Courts are Left to Pick Up the Pieces." *The Times*, June 18.

Faubion, James D. and Jennifer A. Hamilton. 2007. "Sumptuary Kinship." *Anthropological Quarterly* 80 (2): 533–59.

Franklin, Sarah. 2013. *Biological Relatives: IVF, Stem Cells and the Future of Kinship*. Durham: Duke University Press.

———. 2014. "Analogic Return: The Reproductive Life of Conceptuality." *Theory, Culture & Society* 31 (2–3): 243–61.

Hoeyer, Klaus and Linda F. Hogle. 2014. "Informed Consent: The Politics of Intent and Practice in Medical Research Ethics." *Annual Review of Anthropology* 43: 347–62.

Howell, Signe. 2006. *The Kinning of Foreigners: Transnational Adoption in a Global Perspective*. New York and Oxford: Berghahn Books.

———. 2009. "Adoption of the Unrelated Child: Some Challenges to the Anthropological Study of Kinship." *Annual Review of Anthropology* 38 (October): 149–66.

Jasanoff, Sheila. 2005. *Designs on Nature: Science and Democracy in Europe and the United States*. Princeton, NJ: Princeton University Press.

Labassee v. France. Application no. 65941/11. Council of Europe: European Court of Human Rights, June 26, 2014.

Landecker, Hannah. 1999. "Between Beneficence and Chattel: The Human Biological in Law and Science." *Science in Context* 12 (1): 203–25.

Marks, Nicola J. 2017. "Population, Reproduction and IVF in New Caledonia: Exploring Sociocultural and Caring Dimensions of Sustainable Development." *PORTAL Journal of Multidisciplinary International Studies* 14 (2): 6–26.

Mennesson v. France. Application no. 65192/11. Council of Europe: European Court of Human Rights, June 26, 2014.

Modell, Judith. 2002. *A Sealed and Secret Kinship: The Culture of Policies and Practices in American Adoption*. New York and Oxford: Berghahn Books.

Nash, Catherine. 2002. "Genealogical Identities." *Environment and Planning D: Society and Space* 20 (1): 27–52.

———. 2004. "Genetic Kinship." *Cultural Studies* 18 (1): 1–33.

Rose, Nikolas. 2009. *The Politics of Life Itself: Biomedicine, Power, and Subjectivity in the Twenty-First Century*. Princeton, NJ: Princeton University Press.

Strathern, Marilyn. 1992. *After Nature: English Kinship in the Late Twentieth Century*. Cambridge: Cambridge University Press.

———. 1996. "Potential Property: Intellectual Rights and Property in Persons." *Social Anthropology* 4 (1): 17–32.

———. 2005. *Kinship, Law and the Unexpected: Relatives are Always a Surprise*. Cambridge: Cambridge University Press.

Thompson, Charis. 2005. *Making Parents: The Ontological Choreography of Reproductive Technologies*. Cambridge, MA: MIT press.

Van Loon, Hans. 1990. Report on Intercountry Adoption, Prel Doc No 1 of April 1990—Proceedings of the Seventeenth Session, Tome II, 11–119.

van Wichelen, Sonja. 2017. "Reproduction Across Borders: Kinship Legalities in the Bioeconomy." In *Bioeconomies, Life, Technology, and Capital in the 21st Century*, edited by Vincenzo Pavone and Joanna Goven, 207–26. London: Palgrave Macmillan.

———. 2019. *Legitimating Life: Adoption in the Age of Globalization and Biotechnology*. New Brunswick: Rutgers University Press.

Waldby, Catherine and Robert Mitchell. 2006. *Tissue Economies: Blood, Organs, and Cell Lines in Late Capitalism*. Durham: Duke University Press.

Watt, Horatia Muir. 2011. "Private International Law Beyond the Schism." *Transnational Legal Theory* 2 (3): 347–428.

Yngvesson, Barbara. 2010. *Belonging in an Adopted World: Race, Identity, and Transnational Adoption*. Chicago: University of Chicago Press.

Chapter 8

"Stop Thai Women's Wombs from Becoming the World's Womb"

Reproductive Nationalism and the Closure of Commercial Surrogacy in Thailand

Andrea Whittaker

In many societies surrogacy remains a practice not fully understood nor accepted as a means of forming a family.[1] Many nations ban all forms of surrogacy, either "traditional surrogacy" in which a woman uses her own ovum to conceive and gestate a child for other people to parent or "gestational surrogacy" in which in vitro fertilization (IVF) techniques are used to create an embryo which is then inserted and gestated in a surrogate who has no biological relationship to the embryo. Commercial surrogacy is available in some states of the United States, Ukraine, Georgia and Kenya. It is also practiced in some states which lack any regulations. A few other countries such as Australia, Canada, and the United Kingdom allow "altruistic" surrogacy only or allow limited forms of compensation. The restrictions upon surrogacy across the world mean that there is demand for access to such services from intended parents requiring surrogacy to form their families. Until recently, an international commercial surrogacy trade existed in India and many foreign couples sought to access readily available and affordable services there. The trade extended across the region, taking advantage of the lack of legislation at that time in Nepal, Thailand, and Cambodia. These nations have subsequently banned commercial surrogacy and restricted foreigners from seeking surrogacy.[2] In this chapter I examine in detail the events leading to the closure of international surrogacy arrangements in Thailand. Two cases in particular led to the introduction of legislation banning commercial surrogacy in Thailand from July 30, 2015: the notorious

Baby Gammy case in which a baby with Down syndrome was alleged to have been abandoned by his Australian parents and left with his birth mother to raise and a serial surrogacy case involving a Japanese entrepreneur Shigeta Mitsutoki who had entered into surrogacy arrangements with several Thai women to produce over a dozen children.[3] Although extensive media coverage described both cases, and researchers have examined the reporting of these cases in the international media (Riggs and Due 2017; Cohen 2015), there has been no academic work examining how these cases were depicted within the Thai press. In this chapter I explore Thai reactions to both cases. Regardless of the facts of each case, I argue that reactions in the Thai press and online commentary are framed by several cultural understandings about motherhood, Buddhist beliefs, and a pervasive reproductive nationalism. I start with brief summaries of the two cases and then explore Thai reactions. I focus upon these cases not only as a means of examining the issue of surrogacy but also as a lens upon broader sociocultural and political concerns in Thailand.

A number of authors describe the gendering of nationalism and the ways in which men and women differ in their subject positions as citizens and privileged signifiers of national and ethnic boundaries (Kandiyoti 1991; Ram and Jolly 1998; Anthias and Yuval-Davis 1989; Yuval-Davis 1996; Smyth 2017; Whittaker 2004). A prime example is Susan Martha Kahn's (2000) study of the articulation of assisted reproduction to the values and continuity of the Israeli state. Likewise, Lisa Smyth's work on antiabortion politics in Ireland describes the influence of the politics of national identity, and how it reproduces Irishness in traditional familial, patriarchal, and conservative Catholic terms. In Southeast Asia, Aihwa Ong and Michael Peletz (1995, 1) note the articulation of gender with power, nationalism, and capitalism and how "different forms of knowledge and power focus on bodies and sexualities as the crucial sites of political economic and cultural transformations" (see also the discussion of "repronationalism" by Franklin in this volume).

Within Thailand the state has long been involved in the control of women's reproductive bodies through its family planning programs which define which citizens are "fit" to reproduce. Yet the individual actions of women to control their reproduction through abortion are banned and women who abort are depicted as unnatural, un-Thai, and non-Buddhist (Whittaker 2004). In my previous work on debates over abortion regulation in Thailand I noted the importance of women's reproductive bodies as symbolizing the boundaries of the Thai nation (Whittaker 2004, 66–90). Threats to the integrity of women's reproductive bodies were depicted as threatening the values and continuity of a reified Thai culture and racialized identity which stands in opposition to what are depicted as Western values. Rhetoric surrounding the issue of rights to abortion decries the so-called Western values of "free sex" and the lack of respect for the sanctity of life. Women are depicted as requiring protection from such forces to preserve the Thai family and way of life.

Women's participation in Thai society continues to be defined through their reproductivity, with a celebration of maternity and motherhood inherent to public discourse. Although assisted reproduction has become widely accepted in Thai society (Whittaker 2015), surrogacy and the events that unfolded in 2015 have become a new focus for anxieties over biological reproduction and the reproduction of Thai cultural and political values.

POLITICAL CONTEXT IN THAILAND

The surrogacy cases described in this chapter took place against a backdrop of serious political divisions and instability in Thailand. On May 22, 2014, the military staged a coup, led by General Prayut Chan-ocha, and established a military regime headed by the National Council for Peace and Order (NCPO). Thailand is riven with political division between supporters of the former prime minister Thaksin Shinawatra who was ousted in a coup on September 19, 2006, and remains in exile (red shirts) and those opposed to the Shinawatra government (yellow shirts). These divisions have become bound up with rural/urban and class divides and anxieties over the future of the Thai monarchy. A series of violent political protests and counter-demonstrations punctuated several attempts to form a stable government in Thailand. The crisis preceding the 2014 coup followed protests against the popularly elected Pheu Thai Party government of Prime Minister Yingluk Shinawatra (the sister of Thaksin Shinawatra). She dissolved Parliament on December 9, 2013, to force an election, but remained as caretaker prime minister. On May 7, 2014, the Constitutional Court of Thailand found her guilty of charges of abuse of power and removed her from office (*Bangkok Post* 2014a). A few weeks later, the NCPO established a military government, and vowed to conduct national "economic, social and political" reform to fight corruption and ban illegal activities before the next elections were to be held (*Bangkok Post* 2014b).

Since the coup, the NCPO has pursued an agenda with an emphasis on public morality and a crackdown on activities deemed illegal, immoral, or unpatriotic.[4] The social interventions by the NCPO government emphasize Thai nationalism and Thai national values.[5] Within this context, when the Baby Gammy and Shigeta cases emerged, they became a focus for the NCPO in pursuing its agenda of public morality.

METHODS

This work is based on research undertaken for a larger project on international surrogacy in Southeast Asia. All major Thai newspapers and two major Thai language news and social media sites www.kapook.com and www.pantip.com were searched for the period of 2014–2015 using the search terms "surrogacy," "Baby Gammy," and "Shigeta." These were then translated with the assistance of a Thai research assistant. I do not include any identifying information when quoting translations of the Thai online comments to avoid the potential tracking of commentators. No private sites were entered for this information; all are public sites. Only in the case of newspapers citing public figures are real names used. No claim is made as to the representativeness of these views. Rather, they allow insight into the cultural framing of understandings of surrogacy in Thailand at that time.

THE BABY GAMMY CASE

Of all the stories about surrogacy in Thailand in 2014, the story of Baby Gammy drew the greatest amount of worldwide attention to the international surrogacy industry in Thailand and the potential consequences of the industry for the children, surrogate mothers, and parents involved. Baby Gammy and his twin sister were born in Thailand in December 2013 to 21-year-old surrogate mother Pattaramon Chanbua (Goy). On July 4, 2014, in a story in the Thai press, Pattaramon urged Thai women not to become involved in surrogacy and not to treat babies as objects. The article explained that Pattaramon had agreed to engage in surrogacy to pay off family debts and had refused an (illegal) abortion when it was discovered that one of the twins she was carrying had Down syndrome (*Kapook* 2014a). According to Pattaramon, rather than institutionalize the boy child, she offered to care for him herself. The intending parents took the twin daughter and left the country, leaving the son with the birth mother (Murdoch 2014a).

Once the story broke in Australia, the media quickly identified 56-year-old David Farnell and his wife Wendy (formerly Weylu Li) from the Western Australian (WA) town of Bunbury as the couple involved. A media frenzy followed with a series of newspaper articles and television interviews vying for details of the case (Jabour and Foster 2014; Pearlman and Forgan 2014; *Canberra Times* 2014). Investigation by the media revealed that David Farnell had formerly been convicted and served three years' imprisonment for twenty-two child sex offenses against three young girls under 13 in the 1980s (Orr 2014; Kohlbacher 2014).

The public reaction in both Thailand and Australia was vociferous and condemnatory and commentators called for the enforcement of bans against international surrogacy (Ekman 2014; Mitchell 2014; Wilson 2014). An appeal set up on Facebook in August 2014 to raise funds for the future care of Baby Gammy received over 6,000 donations (*Kapook* 2014b). The charity Hands Across the Water was asked to manage the money for the future care of Gammy. Baby Gammy remains in the care of Pattaramon (Hawley 2015).

THE SHIGETA SERIAL SURROGACY CASE

Shortly after the Baby Gammy case, in August 2014, another story broke in the Thai media. It concerned a Japanese man, Shigeta Mitsutoki, the then 24-year-old son of a Japanese billionaire who had reportedly fathered more than a dozen babies to multiple surrogate mothers in Thailand and had fled the country to Cambodia with at least three of the babies (Rawlinson 2014). This case prompted descriptions of Thailand as a "baby factory" in the Thai press. A raid on a Bangkok condominium on August 5 identified nine babies living with nine nannies (Olarn and Whiteman 2014). It was revealed that Shigeta had fathered more than a dozen children through nine surrogate mothers. Staff at one clinic he used, the New Life Clinic, grew suspicious and stopped working with Shigeta after two women got pregnant and he requested more surrogacy agreements. The CEO of that clinic was reported in the press as stating: "He said he wanted 10 to 15 babies a year, and that he wanted to continue the baby-making process until he's dead" (Halpin 2014). She claimed that the clinic had contacted INTERPOL about the case at the time, although INTERPOL claimed to have no record of such a report.

Blurry CCTV images were the only photographs of the "elusive" Shigeta, who was reportedly in Cambodia. In contrast, the Thai doctor involved in the case caught the full force of Thai media attention as he attended Court to give testimony. Surrogate mothers involved in the case also appeared as witnesses, but generally remained anonymous. One surrogate mother's testimony was featured in a press report of the case in *Thairath* newspaper on August 14, 2014, in which one woman claimed she would not go through it again (*Thairath* 2014a). The 32-year-old woman lived in a slum community in Bangkok. The ill-health of her late father had left the family in debt and facing eviction from their rented shack. When her sister came across an advertisement offering US$10,000 for surrogacy, she contacted the agency. Following a complicated pregnancy, she gave birth in June 2013. She described Shigeta as "indifferent" over the birth of the child when she met him for the first time at the New Life Clinic when she signed a document granting him sole custody of the baby.

Shigeta was not charged with any offense (*Thairath* 2014b; Thongnoi and Halpin 2014). He stated through his lawyer that he simply wanted a big family and demanded custody of his children. Although he was summoned by Thai authorities, he did not return to Thailand and was represented by his lawyer. Twelve of the babies were being cared for by Thai social services, with visits allowed by their birth mothers. Shigeta was granted paternal rights over three of the babies by the Central Juvenile and Family Court—a decision that came after a lawsuit against the Social Development and Human Security Ministry for violating Shigeta's rights by taking away his children. Thai media has also reported that Shigeta was believed to have fathered three more babies in India before commercial surrogacy was shut down there (*Khao Sod* 2014a). The All IVF Clinic which had arranged the Thai surrogacies was closed pending investigation (Gecker and Doksone 2014; Murdoch 2014b). Dr. Pisit Tantiwattanakul, the doctor involved, has had his case for indictment delayed four times (*Bangkok Post* 2015).

PUBLIC REACTIONS IN THAILAND

The Thai media and public expressed shock over the Baby Gammy case and the Shigeta "serial surrogacy" case. As I describe below, commentary about the cases deployed discourses on Buddhist ethics, gender, "race," and nationalism and prompted concerns over threats to Thailand's international image and reputation. The mobilization of these discourses not only follows long-standing concerns in Thailand but also provides a further example of the ways in which women's bodies and reproduction are used to represent and constitute different visions of the nation.

Buddhist Ethics

Elsewhere I have documented how societal attitudes toward surrogacy in Thailand have changed over time from initial fear and mistrust to a gradual acceptance (Whittaker 2015). In Thailand the term used for surrogacy, *umbun*, literally means "carrying merit." This refers to beliefs that through the suffering and self-sacrifice of pregnancy and birth a woman achieves Buddhist merit with positive karmic consequences for her reincarnation. As I document in this chapter, this image of surrogacy as a positive and meritorious act was tarnished by the publicity surrounding these two events. This revealed the vulnerabilities produced by an unregulated commercial market in Thailand. A *Thairath* headline played with the term *umbun*, suggesting that rather than "carry merit" surrogacy might "carry demerit" or sin (*umbap*) (*Thairath* 2014c). On social media most people saw the entire arrangement and alleged abandonment as sinful. Many praised Pattaramon for fearing the sin of abortion, whereas bad karma would ensue for the Australian couple. This was stated very bluntly in the following post: "The Thai mother is so generous. May the baby with Down syndrome bring good things to her for the rest of her life. Meanwhile, the Aussie parents will surely get the karma they deserve" (July 4). This implicit contrast between the Buddhist ethics of the birth mother and the intended parents followed a post on the *Kapook* site: "I guess foreigners don't care about sins or merits; but think about how much compassion the surrogate mother has that she didn't abort the baby. Her heart is so noble" (July 4). Other members of the public depicted all parties involved as mercenary and having sinned against the child who was born. A post on *Kapook* from a person calling themselves *Khon Thai* (Thai person) stated: "it shouldn't be called *umbun* [carrying merit] since it is done for money. If it's truly *umbun*, then there shouldn't be any profits involved. That'd actually be considered *umbun*."

As I noted in my earlier work on IVF in Thailand (Whittaker 2015), an early narrative was of Thai cultural and religious values under threat from technology. Such concerns arose again in response to the controversies in 2014. On August 18, 2014, in the newspaper *Matichon*, Chalermpol Polmook expressed unease with technological intervention in conception: "Is such unordinary type of pregnancy a divine wish? Can *karma* be designed by the intelligence of capable humans?" He described a range of ethical issues arising from assisted reproduction more generally, including,

> the selection of specific sperm and eggs for fertilization; whether the left-out embryos get destroyed or used for other purposes; whether such destruction is considered *panatipata* [the destruction of life]; or whether the using of gametes from an unmarried man and woman is considered a violation of the third ethical precept, which forbids sexual misconducts, according to Buddhist teachings. . . . (Polmook 2014)

Likewise, an editorial in *Naewna* newspaper entitled the "The Hidden Sins in the Circle of Surrogacy" (2014c) described a range of ethical concerns raised by the events stating:

> It [surrogacy] stands within the same grey area as "abortion," "organ trade," and "sex trade," in the sense that some people view it as acceptable and some don't. Some think it's the rights of those involved to decide what happens to their life and body. Others see it as a sin, a defiance of God, an act of human trafficking, a sale of bodies, or a destruction of humans' dignity. Moral debates

> surrounding the issue include whether surrogacy is sinful since it involves the creation, rather than the destruction, of a life; where the value of motherhood lies; whether motherhood could be bought and sold; whether the act of using someone else's womb has moral consequences; whether the buying and selling of babies is wrong if surrogacy is not; whether surrogacy should be considered as the separation of a child from his/her mother; whether surrogacy would prompt conflicts in the lives of the parties involved; whether renting someone else's vagina (having intercourse), or any other body parts, is wrong if renting someone else's womb is not; whether organ trafficking is wrong if surrogacy is not; whether it is an exploitation of poor people, who enter surrogacy deals due to financial needs; whether surrogacy should be considered as human trafficking, etc.
>
> So, are there sins hidden in the circle of surrogacy? (*Naewna* 2014)

The ethics of the medical profession were also raised. In his column Chalermpol Polmook questioned who should take responsibility for children born through surrogacy: "an incompetent but greedy obstetrician provides a commercial surrogacy service, but the child born from the service turns out to be disabled, who would be responsible for it? Which agency would volunteer to take the difficult-to-deny responsibility?" (Polmook 2014). Such imagery of a greedy and incompetent medical professional stands in marked contrast to early depictions of Thai IVF doctors as heroes, manipulating high tech interventions to enable infertile couples to form a family. Instead, accusations of multiple clinics breaching Medical Council of Thailand regulations and revelations of the money made from the surrogacy trade presented a different image, epitomized in images of previously privileged and successful doctors appearing before the police.

Gender and Motherhood

The events also prompted comments raising gendered notions of motherhood. These concentrated upon the figure of the gestational surrogate mother. The Baby Gammy case was one of the first in which a Thai woman who had engaged in surrogacy was publicly identified and interviewed. Reports of surrogacy prior to this tended to give anonymous quotes from those who had engaged in surrogacy or secondhand accounts. Pattaramon was initially portrayed sympathetically as a caring, hardworking poor young woman who had been misled and deceived. At first, she was described as "virtuous" and "noble," consistent with Thai valorization of motherhood and nurturing as a normative feminine role bringing Buddhist merit (*bun*) to women. In contrast, the Australian parents were described on social media as "sinful" and "vile."

These initial reactions to Pattaramon's story positioned her within Thai discourses of a good mother. Her claim to have refused to undertake an abortion affirmed the Buddhist value of not taking life and her act of carrying a child for others was seen in terms of self-sacrifice bringing merit. An article in *Kapook* on August 2, 2014, provoked public comments from '*Noonid*' who described Pattaramon as noble: "You have a much nobler heart than the husband and wife do. You carried a child for them. Once the kid has been born with abnormalities, they abandoned the responsibility, but you've decided to continue taking care of him. Your heart is much nobler than theirs" (*Kapook* 2014b).

This sentiment was repeated in another anonymous posting on the same date:

> You are such a noble mother. I've followed this news from the beginning. I already adored you for not aborting the child. And when the real parents didn't take him when he was born with Down syndrome, but you still keep on raising him—that shows that you're his mother. The good deeds that you've done for him [have] brought good fortune. (*Kapook* 2014b)

Revelations that the father of Baby Gammy had been convicted of sex offenses brought condemnation. A posting by '*Ooieng*' on *Kapook* on August 6, 2014, stated: "Both sides are wrong. They're equally vile. The karma has fallen to the child. And the father has been convicted for sexually abusing girls. What's the fate of the girl he has taken with him?"

Most Thai social media posts on the *Kapook* site and commentators in the press concentrated on the role of the Thai surrogate rather than the parents. Thai public attitudes shifted once it was revealed that Pattaramon herself had been acting as a recruiter for surrogacy (*Kapook* 2014c). On August 7, 2014, the Thai newspaper *Kom Chad Luek* reported what it claimed were posts on her Facebook page on May 16, 2014, and April 25, 2014, calling for sperm or egg donors, and offering between 20,000 and 50,000 baht in cash (US$670–1,670) for the genetic material. In an interview, Pattaramon admitted that she recruited for a while but had given it up, and refused to make any further comment. Her involvement in recruiting is not surprising as it was common practice for recruitment to follow social networks. This, however, discredited her image as a poverty-stricken victim and disrupted simplistic characterizations of the industry as one in which those who engage in surrogacy had little or no agency.

A later interview with Pattaramon and her husband in which she described the fundraising money she had received and her intent to buy a house further damaged her image in the press. Following a TV interview in which she described her version of events, several postings to the *Kapook* site on August 5, 2014 questioned her pecuniary motives. The following post was typical: "Going on TV to get donation of 6 million—is this what we call a good person? She's making a living off the child. The foreigners did it because they wanted kids. They were willing to spend their money. Go watch and listen carefully to the surrogate mother. She speaks as if she wants more money."

One *Bangkok Post* commentary described her as a "gold-digging *som tam* seller" (Kolbe 2014). *Som tam* is papaya salad which is a popular food stall item, typically associated with the poorer northeast region of Thailand—an image that carries negative gendered and ethnic connotations.

In contrast with portrayals of Pattaramon, in the Shigeta case, Shigeta Mitsutoki was portrayed as a wealthy, weird recluse. Speculations over why a single man would commission multiple surrogates to produce a large number of children included suspicions of baby selling or organ trafficking. His apparent indifference to the children, leaving them in the care of nannies, reinforced the "unnatural" nature of the scheme and contrasted with the nurturing expected of families.

Racialized Narratives and Surrogacy

Racialized narratives were evoked in Thai media reports of both cases. The image evoked was that of wealthy foreigners (*farang*) coming to Thailand to exploit Thai women's bodies—a sensitive issue in Thailand given its history as a former so-called Rest and Recreation (R & R) destination during the Vietnam War and subsequent development as a sex tourism destination. The public debate over surrogacy once again evoked an image of Thai women's bodies as symbolic boundaries of the nation being breached by foreign forces. Throughout the debates over surrogacy, "Thai" values were described in opposition to "Western" values. On August 7, Pradit Wanarat, member of the National Legislative Assembly (NLA) and president of the National Institute of Development Administration (NIDA), stated on Nation TV that he "personally disagreed with legalizing commercial surrogacy in the Thai society, as it differed from Western societies, and such form of surrogacy would likely lead to further social issues" (*Nation TV* 2014).

"Race" was implicated in descriptions of Baby Gammy as a *farang* (foreign) child. In particular, his white skin indexed his foreignness. In an interview following Gammy's first birthday, Pattaramon was reported as saying that Gammy's white skin draws attention within her community. Pale skin is highly valued in Thailand as a sign of beauty, but in this case it relegates the baby to the status of an outsider. Pattaramon stated that she tells people he is an albino to avoid having to explain the situation. In counterpoint to this, in the final part of the profile of Gammy his grandfather was quoted as stating, "He [Gammy] loves the national anthem and stands still and tall in his walker when it comes on" (Gusmaroli 2015). With this statement the grandfather refers to the practice of publicly broadcasting the national anthem in Thailand every morning and evening, during which the Thai public is expected to stop and stand to attention in respect. Such a statement, whether true or not, signifies Gammy as inherently Thai and patriotic, and a good Thai citizen. Hence, representations of "race," whiteness, disability, and nation were all evoked in this portrait of Gammy.

Likewise, throughout the Shigeta case, Shigeta was referred to as the "Jap" (ยุ่น) father, rather than the more polite term "Japanese" (ญี่ปุ่น). The newspaper *Naewna* on August 15, 2014, declared: "World in Shock as Jap [sic] Man Continues to Hire Surrogate Women as Part of Plan to Father 1,000 Children, Ignores Protests" (*Naewna* 2014a). This was followed by an even more graphic headline on August 16:

> Japanese Media: Surrogate Father Hires 10–15 Thai Women per year to Pump Out "1,000" Babies, Holds Passports of Over 10 Countries—Metropolitan Police to Issue Arrest Warrant, Search Another Illegal Clinic in Sathorn Area. (*Naewna* 2014b)

Thailand has had a vexed history in terms of its relationship with Japan; and Japanese criminal elements have long been involved in the trafficking of women and children for sexual exploitation (Jones et al. 2011). This mistrust emerged in the ways in which Shigeta was depicted. The *Bangkok Post* on August 16, 2014, featured a cartoon by artist 'Dinhin' depicting Shigeta as a stereotypical Japanese with the rising sun bandana around his forehead evoking the Second World War occupation of Thailand. Across his shoulder he carries a sack full of Thai babies while a long arm entitled NCPO attempts to stop him fleeing. In this image, Thai women and babies stand for the Thai nation being exploited while the arm of the Thai military NCPO stretches out to protect and gather up the children. This case further highlighted the use and abuse of Thai women by foreigners.

BRINGING THE IMAGE OF THAILAND INTO DISREPUTE

The various controversies discussed in this chapter shed public light on practices that had been going on in Thai clinics for a number of years. As the quote above reveals, many were concerned that the Baby Gammy case had brought the image (*phap-phot*) of Thailand into disrepute. As one social media report on *Kapook* quoting a Medical Council of Thailand official stated, "Now the more they dig, the more terrible things they find. This has hurt the country's reputation." *Thairath* newspaper described concerns in an article entitled "Surrogacy and the image of Thailand" (อุ้มบุญกับภาพลักษณ์ไทย)

(*Thairath* 2014d) in which the NCPO expressed the view that this issue had damaged the country's reputation abroad and threatened Thailand's medical travel industry—hence action was necessary. This refers to Thailand's status as an economically important hub for medical travel. The term "image" used here refers to two Thai concepts, *phap-phot* and *phap-lak*, which denote notions such as the "(good) name," "standing," "reputation," and "public image" of an institution. Peter Jackson (2004, 186) observes that these terms reflect pervasive cultural concerns with the idea of "face" (*na*) and "reputation" (*cheu-siang*), and the need to "construct positive images" (*sang phap-phot thi di*) and avoid damage to one's reputation. He describes the separation between the public image and what goes on in private in Thailand as a "Thai regime of images" in which the policing of external appearances, performances, and public discourses is foremost and considerable effort is undertaken to expel unwanted representations from the public domain.

In the case of commercial surrogacy, for many years surrogacy arrangements took place quietly and discreetly in clinics—as an unspoken public secret. With the closing down of options for gay couples in India in 2012, a number of international agencies moved operations and new clinics sprang up in Thailand openly advertising commercial surrogacy and ovum donation, targeting gay couples in particular. The damaging publicity that came with the growing number of controversies made commercial surrogacy visible, disrupted the public appearance of Thailand and challenged public expressions of appropriate moral behavior.

THE NCPO ACTS: THE INTRODUCTION OF NEW LEGISLATION

The international embarrassment caused by these events pressured the NCPO to act in keeping with its public morality campaigns. On July 22, 2014 twelve Thai IVF clinics involved in surrogacy that were believed to have breached the Medical Council of Thailand guidelines were shut down. Thai authorities prevented Australian couples from leaving the country with babies born through surrogacy arrangements (*Age* August 11, 2014). There were calls for the introduction of legislation to regulate the industry. Samart Mangsang, who is a leader within the conservative royalist and pro-NCPO People's Alliance for Democracy (PAD), wrote an opinion piece entitled "The sins from surrogacy: An expensive lesson" which called for government intervention:

> Judging from recent developments, it could be argued that the hiring of Thai surrogate women by foreigners is no longer a minor issue that the Thai

> government can ignore, but rather a major national issue worth exploring and setting regulations to prevent further troubles. (Mansang 2014)

Likewise, the editorial of *Khao Sod* newspaper on August 21, 2014, called for the government to enact legislation and clarify the situation, "The entity that could make the issue clear, which will benefit the country, is the government. It can signal when laws would be enacted and what they would entail" (*Khao Sod* 2014b).

Not all commentators called for the banning of surrogacy. Some, such as an editorial in *Kom Chad Luek* (2014), suggested that the industry should be regulated and suggested that a well-regulated international surrogacy industry could be a financial benefit to Thailand:

> "Surrogacy" could perhaps provide good opportunities for Thailand, as our healthcare industry, including prenatal care up until delivery, is considered to have a good standard. We just need to have clear legal procedures or exceptions for it. . . . Legal loopholes must be closed, while opportunities should be open for foreigners to seek the service legally and without stepping into the scope of human trafficking or rights violations. It is a chance for Thailand to become a hub for this field. (*Kom Chad Luek* 2014)

On September 15, the Social Development and Human Society Minister Pol. Gen. Adul Saengsingkaew was quoted as declaring that the NCPO would solve issues of surrogacy in military style by establishing a "war room" to monitor and report on social issues (*Thairath* 2015). The NCPO then revived and modified the preexisting draft *Assisted Reproductive Technologies Bill* number 167/2553 that had first been approved by Cabinet in 2010 but had been waiting for debate by successive parliaments. When the military NCPO revived the Bill, it was renamed the *Protection for Children Born Through Assisted Reproductive Technologies Act*, a name that reflects the change in attitude toward assisted reproduction as the focus shifted from the regulation of technologies to the protection against its harms, and was particularly aimed at stopping the international trade. Despite concerns by some NGOs and academic commentators that the new legislation discriminated against members of the LGBTIQ community who might wish to form families, and that there had been inadequate consultation with women's groups (*Thairat* October 2, 2014), the legislation was passed without further changes.

Prior to 2015, commercial surrogacy and the commercial ovum trade had been banned under guidelines issued by the Medical Council of Thailand, but no legislation existed. The 2015 bill enforced the ban on commercial surrogacy and commercial ovum donation and disallowed intermediaries or brokers for surrogacy arrangements. It restricted the eligibility for surrogacy to heterosexual couples (at least one of whom must be Thai) who have been married for at least two years. In addition, it requires surrogates to be female relatives of the couples requesting surrogacy. The passing of the legislation aimed "to stop Thai women's wombs from becoming the world's womb," according to a media statement citing Wanlop Tankananurak, a member of Thailand's National Legislative Assembly (*ABC News* 2015). In doing so the legislation reasserted a heteronormative family as a Thai value and affirmed the boundaries of Thai-ness through citizenship, banning foreigners from utilizing Thai women's bodies.

OUTCOMES OF THE GAMMY AND SHIGETA CASES

On April 14, 2016, Western Australian Family Court chief judge Stephen Thackray released a judgment in the custody dispute over Gammy's sister contesting whether she should be returned to Thailand to the custody of Pattarmon Chanbua who remains the mother under Thai law [Farnell & Anor and Chanbua (2016) FCWA 17] (Family Court of Western Australia 2016). In his investigation of the case, he determined that the Farnells had not abandoned Gammy, and had wanted to keep him, but that at some stage in the pregnancy "it is clear that Mrs Chanbua had fallen in love with the twins she was carrying and had decided she was going to keep the boy." Chief Judge Thackray stated that the Farnells had "suffered great humiliation and enormous stress for things they did not do." Chief Judge Thackray found that, while the Farnells had intended to keep both children, they were aware that Pattaramon was intending to keep at least one of the babies and were concerned that they would not be able to keep their daughter as well. He described Pattaramon as "a poorly educated young woman who felt obliged to honour at least part of the surrogacy bargain" (Family Court of Western Australia 2016, 105). He noted the inevitable misunderstandings that had arisen in the case given the lack of a common language, cultural differences, dependency upon a facilitator and the nature of the surrogacy industry.[6] Chief Judge Thackray decided that it was in the best interests of Gammy's sister to continue to live with the Farnells rather than be placed in the custody of Pattaramon. In contrast to the widespread sensational coverage of the initial story, the findings of the WA Court investigation were briefly reported in the English language newspaper *The Nation* (*Nation* April 15, 2016). Gammy continues to live in Thailand with the Chanbua family.

Thirteen children involved in the Shigeta case remained in the care of the Social Development and Human Security Ministry's child protection center in Nonthaburi after the surrogacy scandal. A further three children born through surrogacy for Shigeta were reported to have been discovered in

Cambodia (*Bangkok Post* 2016). After long legal battles, Shigeta was granted custody of the children (*Japan Times* 2015; Kyodo News 2018).

CONCLUSION

In this chapter I have described Thai perspectives on two pivotal cases which prompted waves of moral panic over international surrogacy in Thailand. These cases revealed to the Thai public the existence of a thriving international surrogacy trade in Thailand and the legal confusions, vulnerabilities, and ethical dilemmas it posed. The role of traditional and new media in shaping perceptions of these cases is noteworthy. Reports in the press and social media ranged from the factual to the hysterical, galvanizing public opinion and catalyzing political responses. The use of social media by all parties involved in the various cases was sophisticated: to lobby for causes, raise money, and control public images and information. Noteworthy, too, was the lack of Thai news coverage of the resolution of these cases—there was little coverage of the Western Australian Family Court's findings regarding the Baby Gammy case, nor the fate of Shigeta's children.

The cases brought IVF doctors and assisted reproduction more broadly into disrepute and positioned surrogacy as something potentially unethical or morally questionable. The revelations involving high-profile doctors and their private clinics found to be in breach of Medical Council of Thailand guidelines eroded the image of doctors in the early days of IVF as skilled, benevolent, and altruistic—in short, as trustworthy for the ethical management of life. More than anything, these cases revealed the exploitative potential of a surrogacy trade that thrives within countries that have few or no regulations in place.

Prior to these cases in 2014 there had already been several cases involving undesirable and even criminal exploitation of women for surrogacy (Whittaker 2018). Legislation had been awaiting parliamentary endorsement for some time and was the result of lengthy consultation over the previous ten years. For a military government already under heavy foreign criticism and scrutiny, the revelations of these two cases further tarnished the image of Thailand and legislation was introduced quickly.

In this chapter I have discussed how Thai public reactions to both cases were informed by broader debates. In Thailand, ongoing gendered concerns around motherhood and women's reproductive capacity as symbolic of the Thai nation have had a long history. Within a society already acutely sensitive about the presence of a large sex trade for foreigners, the threat posed by commercial surrogacy fed into the Thai military government's agenda of upholding moral and social values and concern with the international tarnishing of

Thailand's image. Long-standing xenophobic fears of exploitation by the West and Japan are also evident in the racialized narratives that emerged in the press and social media. The debates signaled ambivalence over changing gender roles and perceptions of motherhood, the impact of global capital and consumerism upon Thai society, and fears of "westernization" eroding Thai cultural values. These were symbolized by the bodies of Thai women who engaged in surrogacy and the vulnerabilities of small babies being traded by foreigners. A consistent theme throughout the history of assisted reproduction in Thailand is its association with nationalist discourse. By reasserting Thai values in the face of corrupt "Western" colonization of Thai women's bodies through surrogacy, the passing of the restrictions on the surrogacy industry asserted the NCPO's emphasis on "Thai values" and protected Thai women's bodies as symbolic boundaries of the Thai state.

NOTES

1. This research was funded by the Australian Government through an Australian Research Council Future Fellowship. Ethical clearance to conduct the project was received from the Monash University Human Research Ethics Committee (HREC) CF13/3158 - 2013001666. I wish to thank Donhathai Sutassanamarlee who assisted with the Thai translations.

2. Within the region India banned surrogacy for gay couples and singles as of July 9, 2012, and for all foreigners as of November 4, 2015; Nepal outlawed surrogacy as of August 25, 2015; Cambodia banned surrogacy as of October 24, 2016. As will be discussed in this chapter, Thailand banned surrogacy from July 30, 2015 (Whittaker 2018).

3. In April 2018 a Western Australian court found that Gammy's family had not abandoned him, and allowed the parents to retain custody of Gammy's twin sister (*ABC News* 2016). After long legal battles, with the birth mothers and with Thailand's Social Development and Human Security Ministry, Shigeta was granted custody of the children (*Japan Times* 2015; Kyodo News 2018).

4. A range of human rights concerns have been raised about the activities of the NCPO government (US Department of State 2015). The matters of concern have included a ban on political gatherings of more than five people; the detention, arrest, and charging with sedition of a range of people who protested against the coup or have been deemed anti-coup; censorship of new and old media, films or written material deemed provocative or offensive; and the charging of a number of people deemed to have offended the monarchy with lèse majesté offenses.

5. As cited by the National News Bureau of Thailand (Thamdee 2014), the twelve Thai values of the junta are as follows: 1. Love for the nation, religions, and monarchy; 2. Honesty, patience, and good intentions for the public; 3. Gratitude to parents, guardians, and teachers; 4. Perseverance in learning; 5. Conservation of Thai culture; 6. Morality and sharing with others; 7. Correct understanding of democracy with

the monarch as head of the state; 8. Discipline and respect for the law and elders; 9. Awareness in thinking and doing things, and following the guidance of His Majesty the King; 10. Living by the sufficiency economy philosophy guided by His Majesty the King; 11. Physical and mental strength against greed; 12. Concern about the public and national good more than self-interest.

6. In his judgement Court chief judge Stephen Thackray wrote:

> "They did not share a common language, and were dependent on third parties to fill them in on what had happened when they were not personally involved in the action. One of the third parties, who had a clear conflict of interest, decided to keep part of the story to himself. Added to this muddle were not only cultural differences, but also differences in the levels of sophistication of the actors. Their ability to recall what happened, and in what order, has been impaired by the anxiety felt for the health of the babies, and by the tensions that arise when a woman's body is rented for the benefit of others and where the unit of exchange is measured in the life of a new human being. It is little wonder that misunderstandings arose along the way." (Family Court of Western Australia 2016, 16)

WORKS CITED

ABC News. 2015. "Thailand Bans Surrogacy for Foreigners in Bid to End 'Rent-a-Womb' Tourism." February 20. http://www.abc.net.au/news/2015-02-20/thailand-bans-surrogacy-for-foreigners/6163810 (Last accessed October 15, 2018).

———. 2016. "Baby Gammy: Surrogacy Row Family Cleared of Abandoning Child with Down Syndrome in Thailand." April 14. http://www.abc.net.au/news/2016-04-14/baby-gammy-twin-must-remain-with-family-wa-court-rules/7326196 (Last accessed September 30, 2018).

Age. 2014. "Parents Turned Back at Airport: Thai Surrogacy-Couples on Tenterhooks as Authorities Invoke Trafficking Laws." August 11.

Anthias, Flora and Nira Yuval-Davis, eds. 1989. *Woman-Nation-State*. London: Macmillan.

Bangkok Post. 2014a. "Yingluck Out, Partial Cabinet Removal." May 7. http://www.bangkokpost.com/learning/advanced/408502/yingluck-court-ruling-due-at-noon (Last accessed January 7, 2018).

———. 2014b. "Prayuth Assigns Duties, Pledges to Pay Farmers." May 23. https://www.bangkokpost.com/news/politics/411423/prayuth-puts-farmers-first 23 May (Last accessed January 14, 2019).

———. 2015. "Surrogacy Doc Indictment Postponed." *Bangkok Post*, January 15. https://www.bangkokpost.com/print/457032/ (Last accessed January 14, 2019).

———. 2016. "3 Babies Linked to Shigeta in Cambodia." June 17. https://www.bangkokpost.com/news/asean/1012197/3-babies-linked-to-shigeta-in-cambodia (Last accessed January 14, 2019).

Canberra Times. 2014. "Editorial: Baby Gammy Shines a Light on a Murky Practice." August 11, 2014. www.canberratimes.com.au/comment/ct-editorial

/baby-gammy-shines-a-light-on-a-murky-practice-20140811-102vvz.html (Last accessed January 7, 2018).

Cohen, Erik. 2015. "Surrogacy as International Business and National Disgrace of Thailand." *Asian Anthropology* 14 (2): 115–32.

Ekman, Kajsa Ekis. 2014. "Ban the Baby Trade Before it Grows Any Bigger." *Weekend Australian*, September 6.

Family Court of Western Australia. 2016. "Farnell & Anor and Chanbua (2016) FCWA 17." In *FCWA 17*, edited by Family Court of Australia. Perth. http://www.familycourt.wa.gov.au/_files/Publications/2016FCWA17anon.pdf (Last accessed January 7, 2018).

Gecker, Jocelyn and Thanyarat Doksone. 2014. "Thai 'Baby Factory' Triggers Interpol Investigation." *Washington Examiner*, August 22.

Halpin, Dane. 2014. "Interpol 'Warned' of Serial Surrogacy." *Bangkok Post*, August 14.

Hawley, Samantha. 2015. "Baby Gammy, One-year-old at Centre of Thai Surrogacy Scandal, Granted Australian Citizenship." *ABC News*. http://www.abc.net.au/news/2015-01-20/baby-gammy-granted-australian-citizenship/6026600 (Last accessed October 15, 2018).

Jabour, B. and B. Foster. 2014. "Child Abuse Convictions of Gammy's Father Prompt Investigation: Australian Child Protection Workers to Check on Wellbeing of Gammy's Sister, as Surrogate Mother Says She Wants Girl Back." *The Guardian*, 5.

Jackson, Peter A. 2004. "The Thai Regime of Images." *Sojourn: Journal of Social Issues in Southeast Asia* 19 (2): 181–218.

Jones, L., D. Engstrom, P. Hilliard, and D. Sungakawan. 2011. "Human Trafficking between Thailand and Japan: Lessons in Recruitment, Transit, and Control." *International Journal of Social Welfare* 20: 203–11.

Kahn, Susan Martha. 2000. *Reproducing Jews: A Cultural Account of Assisted Conception in Israel*. Durham: Duke University Press.

Kandiyoti, Deniz, ed. 1991. *Women, Islam and the State*. London: Macmillan.

Kapook. 2014a. "Surrogate Mother Opens Up about Baby Gammy Case, Implores Public Not to Treat Babies as Objects." แม่อุ้มบุญ เปิดใจกรณีน้องแกมมี วอนอย่าทำเด็กเป็นสิ่งของ. July 4.

———. 2014b. "Generosity Pours in for Down Syndrome Baby after Aussie Mother Leaves Him with Thai Surrogate Woman." น้ำใจหลั่งไหลช่วยเด็กดาวน์ซินโดรม หลังถูกแม่ออสซี่ทิ้งไว้กับหญิงอุ้มบุญชาวไทย. August 2.

———. 2014c. "Baby Gammy Case: Surrogate Mother Found Posting Online to Recruit Surrogate Women." ข่าวอุ้มบุญ น้องแกมมี พบแม่อุ้มบุญเคยโพสต์หาหญิงรับจ้างอุ้มบุญ. August 7.

Khao Sod. 2014a. "Police to Fly to Cambodia to Prove Existence of 3 Surrogate Babies, Summons 'Doctor' of Infamous Surrogacy Clinic." ตร.จ่อบินเขมร พิสูจน์3ทารก เรียกสอบ "คุณหมอ" คลินิกดัง ทำอุ้มบุญ (18 สิงหาคม 2557 ข่าวสด).

———. 2014b. "Editorial: International Surrogacy." บทบรรณาธิการ: อุ้มบุญต่างชาติ. August 21.

Kohlbacher, Sonia. 2014. "Gammy Case: New 'Victim' Emerges from Child Sex Offender's Past." *The Australian*, October 15, 3.

Kolbe, Max. 2014. "Moral Duplicity Takes Centre Stage in Gammy Case." *Bangkok Post*, August 10.

Kom Chad Leuk. 2014. "Editorial: 'Surrogacy–A Case Study of Thailand." บทบรรณาธิการ: 'อุ้มบุญ' กรณีศึกษาของไท. ย 2014. August 13.

Mangsang, Samart. 2014. "The Sins from Surrogacy: An Expensive Lesson." อุ้มบุญได้บาป: บทเรียนราคาแพง. *Manager*, August 18.

Mitchell, Megan. 2014. "Time to Strengthen Our Lax Surrogacy Laws: Opinion THEIR SAY." *Newcastle Herald,* September 30, 11.

Murdoch, Lindsay. 2014a. "Australian Couple Leaves Down Syndrome Baby with Thai Surrogate." *The Age*, August 1.

———. 2014b. "Dreams of Children Shattered as Thailand Closes All IVF Center." *Sydney Morning Herald*, August 10.

Naewna. 2014a. "World in Shock as Jap Man Continues to Hire Surrogate Women as Part of Plan to Father 1,000 Children, Ignores Protests." ช็อกโลก หนุ่มยุ่น จ้างสาวอุ้มบุญ วางแผนมีลูกพันคน- ไม่สนคำค้าน." August 15.

———. 2014b. "Japanese Media: Surrogate Father Hires 10–15 Thai Women per year to Pump Out '1,000' Babies, Holds Passports of Over 10 Countries–Metropolitan Police to Issue Arrest Warrant, Search Another Illegal Clinic in Sathorn Area." สื่อญี่ปุ่นแฉพ่ออุ้มบุญปั๊ม"ทารก"ตั้งเป้าให้ได้"1,000"คน มาจ้างหญิงไทย10-15รายต่อปีชี้ถือพาสปอร์ตกว่า10 ประเทศ บช.น.เตรียมออกหมายจับแล้ว บุกค้นอีกคลีนิคเถื่อนแถวสาทร. August 16.

———. 2014c. "The Hidden Sins in the Circle of 'Surrogacy'?" บาปแฝงในวงจร'อุ้มบุญ'?

Nation. 2016. "Thai Surrogate Baby Can Live in Australia, Family Court Rules." April 15.

Nation TV. 2014. "NIDA President: Surrogacy Laws Inappropriate for Thai Society." อธิการบดีนิด้าค้านกม.อุ้มบุญไม่เหมาะกับสังคมไทย. August 7.

Olarn, Kocha and Hilary Whiteman. 2014. "Nine Babies Seized as Thailand Cracks Down on Suspected Illegal Surrogacy." *CNN*, August 7. http://edition.cnn.com/2014/08/07/world/asia/thailand-surrogacy-raids/index.html (Last accessed January 7, 2018).

Ong, Aihwa and Michael G. Peletz, eds. 1995. *Bewitching Women, Pious Men: Gender and Body Politics in Southeast Asia.* Berkeley: University of California Press.

Orr, Aleisha. 2014. "Gammy: WA Child Protection Department Knew about Farnell's Child Sex Convictions since May." *Bunbury Mail*, September 24.

Pearlman, J. and D. Forgan. 2014. "Australian Couple Deny Leaving Child in Thailand and Taking Healthy Sister." *The Telegraph*, August 5. https://www.telegraph.co.uk/news/worldnews/asia/thailand/11012571/Australian couple deny leaving-child-in-Thailand-and-taking-healthy-sister.html (Last accessed January 14, 2019).

Polmook, Chalermpol. 2014. "Surrogacy: An Alternative Life . . ." อุ้มบุญ : ชีวิตทางเลือก... 18 สิงหาคม 2557 มติชน โดย เฉลิมพล พลมุข. *Matichon*, August 18.

Ram, Kalpana and Margaret Jolly, eds. 1998. *Maternities and Modernities: Colonial and Postcolonial Experiences in Asia and the Pacific*. Cambridge: Cambridge University Press.

Rawlinson, Kevin. 2014. "Interpol Investigates 'Baby Factory' as Man Fathers 16 Surrogate Children." *The Guardian*, August 23. www.theguardian.com/lifeandstyle/2014/aug/23/interpol-japanese-baby-factory-man-fathered-16-children (Last accessed January 7, 2018).

Riggs, Damien and Clemence Due. 2017. *A Critical Approach to Surrogacy*. New York: Taylor and Francis.

Smyth, Lisa. 2017. *Abortion and Nation: The Politics of Reproduction in Contemporary Ireland*. Oxford: Routledge.

Thairath. 2014a. "1 of Surrogate Mothers Opens Up, Claims She Would Not Have Gone through with Surrogacy if She Could Turn Back Time." 1 ในแม่อุ้มบุญ เปิดใจ ถ้าย้อนเวลาได้ ลั่น ไม่ทำ. August 14.

———. 2014b. "Surrogacy and the Image of Thailand." อุ้มบุญกับภาพลักษณ์ไทย. August 16.

———. 2014c. "9 Babies Confirmed as Jap's Offspring as DNA Samples Match." ทารกเป็นลูกยุ่น 'DNA' ตรงกัน. August 21.

———. 2014d. "Surrogacy Must Not Carry Sin." อุ้มบุญต้องไม่เป็นอุ้มบาป. August 25.

———. 2014e. "Discussions Over Surrogacy Bill See Outcry Over Numerous Loopholes, Cut-off of LGBTQ+ from Opportunity." ถกร่าง ก.ม.อุ้มบุญ โวยช่องโหว่เพียบ ชี้ตัดโอกาสเพศหลากหลาย. October 2.

———. 2015. "'Adul' to Establish War Room to Monitor Social Issues." 'อดุลย์' ฉุยผุดวอร์รูมตามติดปัญหาสังคม (15 ก.ย. 2557; ไทยรัฐออนไลน์ 2014. September 15.

Thamdee, Natthaya. 2014. "NCPO Chief to Bring Thai Moral Values to Government." *National News Bureau of Thailand*.

Thongnoi, Jitsiree and Dane Halpin. 2014. "Japanese Mystery Man Leaves a Tangled Trail in Surrogacy Case." *Bangkok Post*, August 17.

US Department of State. 2015. *Country Reports on Human Rights Practices for 2014 Thailand 2014 Human Rights Report 22 July 2015*. Edited by Human Rights and Labor United States Department of State Bureau of Democracy, Washington. www.state.gov/documents/organization/236692.pdf (Last accessed January 7, 2018).

Whiteman, Hilary. 2014. "Anxious Parents Fear for Babies as Thai Military Tightens Surrogacy Laws." *CNN Wire*, August 19.

Whittaker, Andrea. 2004. *Abortion, Sin and the State in Thailand*. London: Routledge Curzon.

———. 2015. *Thai In Vitro: Gender Culture and Assisted Reproduction*. New York: Berghahn.

———. 2018. *International Surrogacy as Disruptive Industry in Southeast Asia*. New Brunswick: Rutgers.

Wilson, Lauren. 2014. "Surrogacy Inquiry Call." *The Advertiser*, October 10, 12.

Yuval-Davis, Nira. 1996. "Women and the Biological Reproduction of 'the Nation.'" *Women's Studies International Forum* 19 (1–2): 17–24.

Chapter 9

Modes of Mobility

Tracing the Routes of Reproductive Travel in the Asia-Pacific Region

Nicola J. Marks, Vera Mackie, and Sarah Ferber

Reproductive technologies and services have impinged profoundly on the relations between—and constitution of—individuals, groups, and nations. This has occurred amid the uncertainties arising in an industry in which human beings and human emotion are both the "means of production" and the intended final product. As the human reproduction industry expands, we increasingly need to think of it in a regional and global frame. Globalization is "a process of intensifying global social inter-relatedness, whereby space and time are compressed and previously separated locations [are] brought into a new proximity" (Eschle 2002, 316).[1] Technologies such as gamete or embryo freezing and ease of air travel mean that reproductive relations are no longer (if they ever were) "domestic," either in the sense of the family home or of the home country (Franklin 2013, 271).

With globalization, not only do money, products, and people move, but so do "signs, symbols [and] representations" (Mackie and Pendleton 2010). In this sense, IVF and other assisted reproductive technologies (ARTs) have always been a part of globalization. ARTs are associated with movements of techno-scientific knowledges, practitioners, and artifacts, of bodies and biological materials, of cultural norms and regulatory discourses, and of capital. ART-related movements are also often characterized by "reproductive stratification" (Colen 1995), whereby those who travel to access reproductive services tend to be wealthier and often from different ethnic backgrounds from those who provide gametes or gestational labor (Whittaker and Speier 2010).

Accessing or providing assisted reproductive services across borders involves complex forms of mobility which can lead to complicated social and legal issues.[2] For individuals, new forms of reproductive mobility both permit reproductive rights to be optimized and new subjectivities to be experienced. Reproductive travel to avoid legal prohibitions in a home jurisdiction can raise questions about individuals' legal autonomy in the pursuit of physical and emotional well-being. There are also significant questions concerning the rights of poor women, of children born into unstable regulatory environments, of LGBTQI or single people, or of those whose rights are seen to have greater or lesser valence because of gender, ethnicity, class, or racialized positioning. For the nation-state, reproductive mobilities affect the capacity of jurisdictions to balance local exigencies—such as activism for more or less liberal laws—with concerns about exploitation or commodification.

In recent years, there has been increasing public and media attention to travel for fertility services in the Asia-Pacific region. Positive stories emphasize the increased choices that are now open to families. A lesbian couple from New Caledonia, for example, was able to access in vitro fertilization (IVF) by traveling to New Zealand, as fertility treatments in their home country are only available to heterosexual couples (Akersten 2009). Other stories highlight controversies, such as an Australian becoming a first-time mother at 62 after traveling overseas to obtain a third-party embryo (Spooner and Carmody 2016), or children allegedly abandoned in Thailand or India by their Australian commissioning parents (Hawley 2015; Whittaker 2016b; Whittaker in this volume; Foreign Correspondent 2015; Murdoch 2017).[3] This highlights the diverse and at times competing interests, rights, and responsibilities involved in reproductive travel.

Under globalization, production, consumption, and reproduction transcend the scale of the nation-state, while institutions of global governance deal—or fail to deal—with issues that go beyond the boundaries of nation-states. For social scientists one of the challenges in this context is to shift from operating in a largely national frame to addressing issues which necessarily cross national borders. We need to be sensitive to questions of scale—from the most intimate embodied experiences to the local, the national, the regional and the global. Mackie and Stevens (2009, 3) argue for the necessity of carrying out micro-level case studies which are embedded in an understanding of global processes.

In this chapter we explore these processes through an examination of the modes and routes of mobility associated with assisted reproduction in the Asia-Pacific region. We first highlight that IVF has always involved movements of people, biological and technical entities, capital, and discourses. We then focus on three selected nodal points: Australia, Japan, and French Polynesia. Each of these nodes is associated with particular, at times intersecting, routes to destinations where reproductive services are available. These case studies highlight that the implications of reproductive mobility in specific cultural contexts require culturally attuned interpretation, to some extent defying the neat categorization of rights and roles.

DIVERSE MOBILITIES

From their earliest development, reproductive technologies were built on transfers of information between medical professionals working in a globalized profession. Although much of the early history of IVF is marked by secrecy and competition to accomplish world "firsts" (Bharadwaj 2002), many scientific developments would not have been possible without international movements of scientists, such as the training of Indian scientists in the United Kingdom or the international workshops at Bourn Hall Clinic, established by Edwards and Steptoe in 1980 (Bharadwaj 2002; Cohen et al. 2005; Leeton 2013). Many ART scientists continue to work across borders. The spread of knowledge between professionals has recently been facilitated by the internet. Patients and commissioning parents, too, communicate with each other over the internet, although the "digital divide" is still an important element of stratification (Clarke et al. 2003, 177–78).

IVF was implemented alongside other technologies developed in multiple sites, and then adopted and adapted in new ones. These technologies include freezing of gametes and embryos, microscopy, laparoscopy, ultrasound, the development of culture mediums, fertilization by microinjection, the micromanipulation of sperm by laser, and genetic diagnosis (Suzuki 2014; Frank 2009). New drugs became commodities in the global pharmaceutical industry. The use of fertility drugs to create multiple ova from a single cycle has also opened up marketing possibilities for IVF and other ARTs, permitting multiple clients, potentially in several different locations, to attain a pregnancy. Freezing technologies have been particularly important as they enable the separation in both space and time of harvesting, fertilization, and implantation, paving the way for current forms of reproductive travel (Franklin 2013, 119).

People and biological material also move internationally for IVF. Would-be parents travel in search of genetic material or gestational labor (often referred to as surrogacy). This scenario was dramatically conveyed in the documentary *Google Baby* (2009), where an Israeli agent purchases oocytes, arranges for fertilization by the sperm of a commissioning father, arranges for the embryo to be implanted in a gestational mother in India, with the baby finally being taken to Israel by the commissioning parents. The tears shed by the gestational mother after relinquishing the baby offer a glimpse into the emotional costs associated with these practices.

These difficulties are also made more visible in extreme circumstances, such as the aftermath of an earthquake in Nepal in 2015. It was revealed that the Israeli government evacuated children but left gestational mothers behind. At that time, Nepal was an important destination for Israelis to make surrogacy arrangements with Indian and Thai women (Kamin 2015). These events can highlight issues of what has been called "reproductive trafficking" (Shalev, Eyal and Samama 2017).

Cross-border reproduction can also involve restrictions on the mobility of some people and biological materials. If oocytes are not to be frozen, fertilization and implantation need to take place with the provider of oocyte(s) and the gestational mother in close proximity. Gestational mothers may be compelled to stay in particular places while they are pregnant with the child intended for commissioning parents. This is part of the way women carrying babies in surrogacy arrangements are disciplined into "perfect mother-workers" (Pande 2010, 2017). Commissioning parents may also be obliged to be on hand to wait for the birth or for legal procedures to recognize their parentage or adoption (Deomampo 2013).

These movements are shaped by cultural norms and regulatory discourses, which also travel and are transformed internationally as part of globalization. Legal scholars from Japan, for example, traveled to Australia to study the social and legal environment for the implementation of new reproductive technologies (Kinjō 1996). Knowledge gained by doctors traveling to Monash University in Melbourne was instrumental in helping to formulate the Tōhoku University charter for IVF and embryo transfer (Suzuki 2014, 188). For Taiwan, with reference to multiple-embryo implantation policies, Wu (2012) identifies complex adaptations of global trends in regulation, variously deployed in debate and practice at the local level.

Changes in regulatory regimes have corresponding effects on the routes of reproductive travel. The enactment of the *Bioethics and Biosafety Law* in South Korea in 2003, or recent legislation to tighten up the regulation of access to reproductive medical services in India and Thailand, have meant that clients seek reproductive medical services in alternative destinations. (In Thailand, the *Protection for Children Born Through Assisted Reproductive Technologies Act* was enacted in February 2015; while in India, The Surrogacy Regulation Bill was passed in December 2018 [Martin 2014; Murdoch 2014; Semba et al. 2010, 350; Government of Thailand 2015; Government of India 2018; Dey 2018; Bhangra 2019; Mohanka in this volume; Whittaker in this volume]). In some cases, the gestational mothers will cross borders into a neighboring country for implantation and then cross back to give birth. Medical professionals also cross borders to facilitate these procedures (Whittaker 2018). New laws and legal differences can form the basis for client choices in the first place as well as leading to problematic outcomes.

Recent controversies concern babies not allowed to leave their birth country with their commissioning parents, babies unable to obtain nationality in their commissioning parents' country, and babies abandoned by commissioning parents due to marriage breakdown, unwillingness to look after more than one twin, or because the child had a disability.[4]

Linguistic or cultural connections may also come into play. One of the attractions of India for anglophone commissioning parents was the ability to interact with medical professionals in English. The common use of the English language in disparate places is one legacy of the history of colonialism. In places like Thailand, although English is not the first language, medical professionals in clinics are often able to interact with international clients in English (Whittaker and Speier 2010). Many clients also make use of brokers who provide access to interpreters, translators, and legal advisors in addition to medical personnel (Sumiyuki International Limited Company undated).

The international movement of capital is central to the IVF industry. Economic inequality comes into play when clients travel to countries where medical services are available more cheaply than in their home countries. International political economy influences which people can purchase reproductive services or genetic material and which people sell them, notwithstanding the supplicatory position sometimes characteristic of those seeking reproductive services.[5]

IVF and ARTs are thus tightly woven into complex movements—as well as restrictions and transformations—affecting scientists, techniques, and scientific publications; biological material (eggs, sperm, embryos); bodies (providers of gametes, commissioning parents, gestational mothers, infertile couples, babies); capital; and regulatory discourses and cultural norms. A range of factors affects how these are shaped at the local and global level. We explore these processes through a discussion of three nodal sites in the Asia-Pacific region: Australia, Japan, and the French Pacific. As we shall see, there is no simple division between "sending" and "receiving" countries. Starting with each nodal point, we can trace some of the routes of reproductive travel in the region, and clarify the factors which shape them.

Based on our case studies concerning reproductive travel in the Asia-Pacific region, we posit several factors associated with the modes and routes of reproductive travel: the existence or lack of regulation, gaps between regulatory regimes in different places, gaps between the availability of particular reproductive medical services in different places, the promotion of medical travel and reproductive travel in particular local sites, economic inequality, linguistic or cultural connectedness, historical connections, diasporic connections, former colonial relationships, and geographical proximity. The significance of these factors for the ways in which assisted reproduction is carried out is in many ways context-dependent, signaling the value of local case studies as a means of characterizing the global dimensions of ARTs.

ROUTES OF REPRODUCTIVE TRAVEL IN THE ASIA-PACIFIC REGION

The Asia-Pacific region is experiencing major growth in the fertility services industry (Report Buyer 2016), and has always been important in the development of reproductive technologies. The first pregnancy from an embryo created *ex utero* was reported in 1973 by De Kretzer et al. (1973) in Australia, although it ended in miscarriage. The first full-term IVF pregnancy and birth in the United Kingdom in July 1978 (Steptoe and Edwards 1978) was closely followed by a birth in India in the same year (Bharadwaj 2002). Other early births through IVF conception occurred in Australia in 1980, the United States in 1981, France, Sweden, and Austria each in 1982, and New Zealand and Japan in 1983 (Suzuki 2014). IVF came to some countries much later. In the Philippines the first baby born through IVF was in 1996 (de Castro and Toledano 2009, 430) and in New Caledonia in 2005 (Les Nouvelles Calédoniennes 2005). Until recently, India and Thailand were popular destinations for reproductive travel although, as noted earlier, the regulatory regimes have changed (Whittaker 2009; Whittaker in this volume; Whittaker 2018; Mohanka in this volume; Pande 2011; Everingham 2014; AAP 2015; Stockey-Bridge 2018). Cambodia and Nepal became popular destinations, before they, too, enforced restrictions (Bhowmick 2016; Barker 2017; Whittaker in this volume).

AUSTRALIA

Australia was a major site for the initial development of assisted reproductive technologies. In addition to the aforementioned first IVF pregnancy, the team at Monash was responsible for the first birth from a pregnancy using a donor egg in 1983 and one of the first births from a frozen embryo in the same year.[6] The early days of IVF were characterized by Australian scientists traveling internationally, sharing their knowledge of cattle reproduction in the United Kingdom (Leeton 2004; Frank 2009) or learning new technical skills in Singapore (Dimoia 2013; Franklin 2007).

This early development of technical expertise, in addition to strong regulation (Leeton 2004; Johnson 2006), accompanied by the professional guidelines of the National Health and Medical Research Council (NHMRC),[7] have been important contributing factors to Australia's place as a world leader in both fertility services and regulatory responses. Despite recent controversies over false hope, fruitless treatments and high costs to individual patients and the national health insurance scheme, IVF is a thriving business (Four Corners 2016). Many clinics also offer their services to international patients (IVF Australia n.d.),[8] while some Australians travel overseas to access reproductive services. This can be to access cheaper services, since cost is an important factor shaping reproductive mobilities (Rodino et al. 2014, 1422–31), as well as to access services not permitted at home, including "social" sex selection (Whittaker 2011).

IVF centers in Australia once offered the option of only implanting embryos of a particular sex, but stopped in 2005 when the NHMRC guidelines explicitly banned sex selection, except to avoid particular sex-linked diseases. This ban has been criticized by some fertility centers (Genea 2013) and resulted in high-profile fertility specialists arguing that sex selection for "family balancing"[9] was unproblematic and that current regulation in Australia "forced" patients overseas (Whittaker 2011, 614; Lateline 2017; Miller 2017).

A Fertility Society of Australia (2013) study suggests that increasing numbers of Australians are traveling overseas to select embryos of a specific sex. This study tracked requests by Australian patients for sex selection at IVF clinic Superior ART, in Bangkok. The results were reported by a fertility doctor working at a joint-venture clinic in Australia called Sydney IVF (now Genea). Part of the attraction of Bangkok's Superior ART clinic for sex selection, in addition to its English language website, was its initial recommendation on Genea's Australian website, in turn, shared on pregnancy discussion boards (BellyBelly 2008). Although Genea was keen to state that they were not "referring" patients (Whittaker 2011, 614), and the original website identified by Whittaker is no longer to be found, this example highlights the international links between fertility providers.[10]

International movements of capital also play a role here since an Australian company invested in a Thai laboratory providing the technique underpinning sex selection (Whittaker 2011, 614). This shows the importance of capital, professional and industrial networks, communication technologies, the increased ease of travel for some patients, and differences in regulation in encouraging reproductive mobilities. With recent tightening of Thailand's IVF-related rules and regulation (nonmedical sex selection was in fact in breach of the Medical Council of Thailand's professional guidelines), Thailand is no longer a popular destination and Superior ART has explicitly distanced itself from offering sex selection, commercial surrogacy, oocytes, and sperm (Whittaker 2016, 71–78; Superior ART 2007).

The strict Australian regulations not only encourage reproductive movements out of Australia but also toward it. Commercial oocytes, for example, are not available in Australia, meaning that they will be sought elsewhere. Companies have chosen to import oocytes from places such as the United States (Stokes 2015). The US women who provide oocytes are not, at least formally, meant to be paid beyond compensation for travel and medical costs but the trade in ova in the United States is widespread (Spar 2007). Another way to address the market for eggs (using fresh rather than frozen eggs) is to fly in the providers. South African women, for example, are offered the "trip of a life time" in exchange for their eggs and living costs during their Australian stay (Dobbin 2016). Such developments highlight the importance of regulatory factors, a trend which has been particularly noticeable in the case of gestational surrogacy.

While the use of IVF is tightly regulated in Australia, the situation is more complicated with respect to surrogacy (Whittaker 2016b). In Australia's federal system there are differences in family law, the regulation of adoption and the regulation of assisted reproduction from state to state (Commonwealth of Australia 2016). Although surrogacy has been decriminalized, it is still seen as an option of "last resort" (Millbank 2012, 102) and is in all cases meant to be "altruistic" (ABC Background Briefing 2017). It is illegal to compensate someone who undertakes surrogacy with any monies other than medical and other out-of-pocket expenses in all states and territories except the Northern Territory. In Queensland, New South Wales, and the Australian Capital Territory the law serves "to discourage residents from engaging in surrogacy in countries where compensating a surrogate for more than medical and out-of-pocket expenses is legal" (Everingham 2014, 68).

The gaps between different states and the ban on commercial surrogacy mean that there is the potential for mobility between states as well as overseas travel in search of gestational surrogates, in particular, as offers of "altruistic" surrogacy in Australia do not match demand (ABC Background Briefing 2017). The first highly publicized case of altruistic surrogacy in Australia was in 1989 (Millbank 2012). It is reported that in 2011, only eighty Australian women offered to carry out altruistic surrogacy (Barlass 2014). In recent years, international surrogacy cases have become more visible and there are documented cases of gay male couples traveling to the United States and other places in order to enter into surrogacy agreements (Miller 2012; Wood 2015; Bastians 2016; Keaney in this volume). Children born of overseas commercial arrangements, however, are not always recognized as the legal children of commissioning parents when they return to Australia (Bailes 217).

Regulation shapes some Australians' choices to travel overseas to access surrogacy and other reproductive services. Commissioning parents may choose to travel to a site where regulation is less stringent than at home (such as India or Thailand until recently) (Foreign Correspondent 2014). Commissioning parents may also choose destinations which have clear enabling regulation. In the US state of Nevada, commissioning parents can be named as parents on the child's birth certificate, meaning there will be fewer problems in bringing a child back to Australia. If the child is genetically related to one of the parents, they can apply for Australian citizenship for the child on the basis of descent (Australian Government Department of Immigration and Border Protection n.d.).

In turn, regulations and legislation are shaped by globalized mobilities and immobilities of people (such as babies caught in an international legal impasse), cultural norms, and ethical discourses. As Whittaker (2016; in this volume) shows for Thailand, public and political discussions of a law covering assisted reproduction began as early as 2000 and the draft "Pregnancy by Medically Assisted Reproductive Technology Act" bill was approved in 2010. The renamed "Protection of Children Born from Assisted Reproductive Technologies Act," however, was not passed until 2015 (Government of Thailand 2015). This law did not become a national priority until the issues of commercial, international IVF and surrogacy became a matter of international controversy (AAP 2015), facilitated by the Thai media painting Thailand as a "baby factory." This was in response to high profile cases such as "Baby Gammy." Another case involved an unmarried Japanese man, Shigeta Mitsutoki, who was reported to have fathered more than a dozen babies in Thailand using gestational birth mothers. After long legal battles, with the birth mothers and with Thailand's Social Development and Human Security Ministry, the man was granted custody of the children (Japan Times 2015; Kyodo News 2018; Whittaker in this volume). These changes in regulations around surrogacy may lead to immobilities, especially when rules are tightened, leaving intending parents and babies stranded overseas (Auerbach 2014; Barker 2017).

JAPAN

Japan, as another relatively wealthy country with a well-developed medical system, has similarities with Australia. There are differences, however, in how reproductive health services are regulated. Very small numbers of children come up for adoption in Japan, partly due to the very low numbers of babies born out of wedlock.[11] In addition to the restrictions set out in the Civil Code of Japan, adoption agencies often impose stringent conditions concerning the age of the adoptive parents, their income, and expectations that one parent would be a full-time career (Noda and Netsu 2011).

Japan, like Australia, has a well-developed reproductive medical industry so there is rarely any need to travel overseas to access "basic" reproductive services such as IVF. In the earliest stages of IVF in Japan, procedures generally involved the genetic material of married couples. The IVF-ET Charter of the Tōhoku University School of Medicine, the first to be codified in Japan in 1983, states that procedures "should not be performed outside of marriage"; that "the patient has ovaries from which mature ova can be collected"; and that "usable sperm can be obtained from the patient's spouse" (Suzuki 2014, 189). The Tōhoku charter was influential as other hospitals started to practice IVF and develop their own guidelines. In subsequent years, artificial insemination by donor sperm has become an accepted practice. Japan has never had legislation concerning such practices as surrogacy, but rather relies on guidelines issued by the medical profession (Ishii 2009; Mackie 2013, 2014a). The Japan Society of Obstetricians and Gynecologists (JSOG) advises its members against facilitating surrogacy agreements. Doctors who perform procedures banned by JSOG risk losing their license to practice medicine. The Japanese Institution for Standardizing Assisted Reproductive Technology permits IVF with donated eggs from a friend or sister (Ishii 2009, 183). The Science Council of Japan (2008) has recommended legislating to prevent surrogacy where profit is involved, but as yet no legislation has been enacted. Only one practitioner in Japan—Netsu Yahiro of Suwa Maternity Clinic—openly facilitates altruistic surrogacy, but only where the surrogate mother is a relative of the intending mother. Early cases involved altruistic surrogacy for a sister or sister-in-law, but Netsu now only facilitates mother-daughter surrogacy (Netsu and Sawami 2009).

For these reasons, some Japanese couples travel overseas to access services such as purchasing ova or engaging in an agreement with a gestational mother. Providers of reproductive services outside Japan now maintain specific Japanese language websites, such as India's Medi Bridge Medical Tourism Agency (Medibridge n.d.). As with Australian commissioning parents, destinations have until recently included India, Thailand, and the United States. South Korea was a destination for some services until the *Bioethics and Biosafety Law* (enacted 2003; effective 2005) prohibited commercial transactions related to third-party gametes (Semba et al. 2010, 350). There is at least one agent in Tokyo who has facilitated cross-border reproductive travel through arrangements with a specific clinic, the Nevada Center for Reproductive Medicine. It can be estimated that the couples from Japan who have entered into surrogacy arrangements overseas number in the hundreds (Mukai 2007, 22).[12]

Some recent high-profile cases illustrate the enmeshment of individuals from Japan in the global reproductive industry. Yamada Ikufumi and Yamada Yuki entered into a surrogacy contract with Pritiben Mehta, who carried an embryo created from an ovum harvested from an anonymous Indian woman and the sperm of Yamada Ikufumi. The Yamadas divorced in June 2008 shortly before Manji was born to the Indian gestational mother on July 25, 2008. Because the Japanese legal system recognizes the birth mother as mother, and the birth mother's husband as father, Yamada Ikufumi was unable to register Manji as his daughter. The Indian legal system at that time did not recognize or regulate surrogacy, and contracting parents would usually adopt children born to surrogate mothers. The Guardians and Wards Act of 1890, however, does not allow single men to adopt girls. Similarly, in Japan, only married couples can carry out special adoption (Mackie 2014a).[13] This precluded the divorced Yamada Ikufumi from adopting baby Manji. The clinic was willing to certify that Yamada was the genetic father, but it was unclear who should be registered as mother, so Manji was without a birth certificate or a passport. Yamada appealed to the Indian government to allow documents to be issued, and the city of Anand issued a birth certificate which just showed Yamada as father. The Indian Supreme Court granted temporary custody to the grandmother Yamada Emiko (Points n.d., 6), and the Rajasthan regional passport office issued an identity document. The document did not mention nationality, mother's name or religion, and was good for just one trip to Japan. The Japanese Embassy issued a one-year visa for Manji on humanitarian grounds. Manji was able to travel to Japan, but was illegitimate and stateless.

In another complex international case, a celebrity couple in Japan, Mukai Aki and her husband Takada Nobuhiro saw Mukai's battle with cervical cancer closely followed by the media. Mukai underwent a hysterectomy but was able to keep her ovaries. The Takadas traveled to Nevada where Cindy Van Reed carried twins conceived from the married couple's sperm and ova. Nevada named the Takadas as parents on the twins' birth certificates and the children had US nationality on the jus soli principle.[14] They were unable to register the children on their return to Japan, but after several years of legal struggle were able to adopt them. They could apply for the naturalization of the children three years from the adoption (Mukai 2002a [2001], 2002b, 2004, 2007).

Because there is no legal regulation of surrogacy in Japan, the Yamadas and the Takadas had not broken any laws. They encountered problems when they tried to register their children because, as noted earlier, the birth mother is considered the mother of a child and the husband of a married woman is considered to be the father. Newborn children are registered in the family register of their parents. Japanese nationality depends on being registered in a family register, so that a child who is not in a family register does not have Japanese nationality. It is likely that most of the Japanese couples who have entered into transnational surrogacy arrangements have been able to register their children without admitting to the surrogacy agreement, for only a small number of cases have ended up in the courts. In the case of the Takadas, however, their surrogacy agreement was public knowledge. Even though they had a birth certificate from Nevada naming them as the parents, the local ward office refused to include the children in their family register and this was upheld in the courts (Mackie 2014a).[15] This highlights the disjunctures between laws and practices in different places around the world.

In another high-profile case, parliamentarian Noda Seiko traveled to the United States to obtain a third-party ovum, after undergoing fourteen rounds of unsuccessful IVF treatment in Japan. The ovum from a US woman was fertilized by Noda's de facto husband's sperm and implanted in Noda's womb. Noda returned to Japan and bore the child. Because Noda was the birth mother there were no problems in registering the child as her own. Nevertheless, there was public controversy because of her age (she was around fifty when she bore the child) and because she had purchased a third party ovum overseas. Noda used the same reproductive travel agency as the Takadas, and her obstetrician was the aforementioned Netsu Yahiro. Noda has become an advocate for reformed adoption procedures and for making assisted reproduction more available in Japan.

Most of the public discourse on reproductive matters in Japan concerns married, heterosexual couples of Japanese ethnicity. There is often a nationalist emphasis as the country deals with a low birth rate and an aging population (Mackie 2014b). Statistics show people marrying later, choosing not to marry, having children later, or not bearing children. There is very little public discussion of the use of assisted reproduction by those outside the system of heterosexual marriage, and in practice most assisted reproductive services are restricted to married couples. Nevertheless, Higashi Koyuki and Masuhara Hiroko have raised the issue of lesbian motherhood in their book *Futari no mama kara, kimitachi e* (To you from your two mothers) (Higashi and Masuhara 2014; see also Ringler 2016), and anecdotal evidence suggests that gay and lesbian parents are finding ways to access assisted reproduction.[16] Special adoption is restricted to married couples; same-sex marriage is not recognized; and this precludes same-sex partners from adopting children. Nontraditional families are often explored in popular cultural forms, though, as has been discussed elsewhere (Mackie 2013, 2014b).

Japan is not the only place where IVF services are targeted at married heterosexual couples. France has a similar heteronormative approach. This influences the French Pacific where reproductive travel needs to be understood in its geographical and historical contexts.

NEW CALEDONIA AND FRENCH POLYNESIA

It is often the case that inhabitants of a colonial metropolis travel to former colonies to access cheaper health services delivered in their own language (as when people traveled from the United Kingdom toward former British colonies like India).[17] In French Polynesia and New Caledonia, however, some women and their partners travel toward metropolitan France to access assisted reproduction, or to other places such as New Zealand. In addition to financial considerations, colonial histories, geographical proximity, and regulatory frameworks play important roles.

New Caledonia and French Polynesia remain in colonial relationships with France despite some increased autonomy. The United Nations lists these countries among those that are non-self-governing and should therefore be decolonized (Wamytan 2005; United Nations 2015). French Polynesia has, since 2004, been called a French Overseas Collectivity (Collectivité d'Outre Mer). It has some say in its governance, in terms of social security provisions, public health, and fiscal policy (loi organique n°2004-192, updated in 2010, with the loi organique n°2010-704). New Caledonia has a special status established through the Noumea Accord of 1998. It is semi-independent and voted in 2018 (in the first of three planned referenda) against independence. New Caledonians manage their own social security provisions, public health, and fiscal policy (Ministère des Outre-Mer n.d.).

France has always had strong pronatalist policies (Löwy 2006). These are translated into financial support for IVF treatment through social security provisions, including up to six free intrauterine implantations of embryos created through IVF (Natisens n.d.; Fivfrance.com 2014). Because they are French citizens, French Polynesians and New Caledonians can access this support in mainland France. Some French policies thus directly encourage the international movement of Polynesians and New Caledonians.

In French Polynesia, the Caisse de Prévoyance Sociale (CPS) (social security insurance fund) is a not-for-profit countrywide compulsory health insurance scheme which reimburses IVF cycles, but five, rather than six, embryo implantations (CPS 2013; Forum Naissance en Polynésie 2012). Because there are no IVF clinics on the islands, those wishing to access fertility treatment must cross borders. The CPS recognizes this and reimburses full medical costs for IVF in France, and partial costs in New Zealand (Forum de FIV. fr. 2017)

In New Caledonia, the Caisse de Compensation des Prestations Familiales, des Accidents du Travail et de Prévoyance des Travailleurs de Nouvelle-Calédonie (CAFAT, New Caledonian compensation fund for family benefits, work accidents and workers' insurance) like the CPS, reimburses IVF costs at a slightly lower rate than metropolitan France. Payments also need to be made up-front by the patients, unlike in France.[18] Since there is a fertility center in the capital Nouméa (Calédo Fertilité), women seeking IVF do not have to travel across borders to access their treatments, but some choose to. Reasons for travel include the closure of Calédo Fertilité in holiday periods and some women's desire not to waste any time accessing treatment (Le Forum de FIV.fr 2014; interview with IVF biologist, June 2016), as well as the local unavailability of specialist services such as pre-implantation genetic diagnosis.

New Zealand remains a popular place to access IVF, as evidenced by the French language brochures offered by New Zealand fertility centers, which make specific mention of both New Caledonia and French Polynesia (Fertility Associates 2014). This stems in part from its geographical proximity to both countries and the frequency of flights. Clients need to weigh up the added medical costs of New Zealand against the longer trip to mainland France, the lack of family support networks in New Zealand, and the need to hire interpreters if they do not speak English (Forum Naissance en Polynésie 2012).

French Polynesia's CPS has medical evacuation arrangements with New Zealand, making it an established destination for medical care. New Zealand is seen as the place to go for many Polynesians wanting IVF, rather than Nouméa, despite the much higher costs of treatment (interview with IVF doctor, June 2016). New Caledonia's CAFAT supports medical evacuation to Australia (arrêté n°2016-243/GNC), but New Caledonians, if they travel in the region for IVF, choose New Zealand rather than Australia (interview with IVF doctor, June 2016) indicating the importance of the centers' advertising and willingness to facilitate French speakers' access to their websites.

New Caledonia and French Polynesia have particularly high costs of living (34 percent higher than in mainland France for New Caledonia and 26 percent higher for French Polynesia). This is due to historical financial and trade arrangements with mainland France leading to protectionist practices, and to the high number of well-paid civil servants from mainland France living on the islands (Roubio Collet 2012; Wasmer and David 2012; Dorney 2013). Long stays in places like New Zealand for fertility treatments are thus not unaffordable, compared to staying at home, especially in capital cities.

Although New Caledonia is a wealthy country, it is also characterized by inequality (Ris 2013, 59–72). Indigenous Kanak peoples under early French settlement in 1853 were displaced on to reserves and prevented from participating in economic life (Zocca 2006, 265–316; Merle 2000). They are less wealthy than New Caledonians of European descent, and tend to live at greater distances from the capital city Nouméa where the fertility center and international airport are located. This colonial legacy can make IVF less accessible to some patients. This is countered, however, by CAFAT reimbursing the cost of medical treatment, as well as flights from remote areas of New Caledonia toward Noumea and local accommodation. Essential, too, is the determination of fertility specialists in Noumea to encourage remote patients to travel to the capital for IVF (interviews with two IVF doctors, June 2016; Ma).

Regulation also encourages fertility travel. IVF in New Caledonia and French Polynesia is regulated by metropolitan France's bioethics law (loi n° 2011–814 relative à la bioéthique, July 7, 2011). Although these two countries can make their own decisions regarding healthcare and social security, they follow mainland France in terms of which procedures are legal. Only certain people from New Caledonia and French Polynesia are supported in their access to IVF and ARTs: those who are in a heterosexual married or de facto couple, where the woman is under 43.

In France, assisted reproduction is explicitly not aimed at being a pathway to "alternative" families (Agence de la Biomédicine 2009). Assisted reproduction was excluded from recent legal changes regarding same-sex marriage (Avril and Gicquel 2013, 171–202).[19] People from French Polynesia and New Caledonia travel to countries with less heteronormative access policies, such as New Zealand (Akersten 2009) or some European countries (interview with IVF doctor, June 2016).

Another restriction relevant to ART access is the strong cultural and legislative opposition to practices thought to encourage commodification of the body, as this is seen to go against public order. Protection of the integrity of the body is enshrined in the French Civil Code (article 16–7) and for assisted reproduction in the loi bioéthique, as has been reiterated by the French justice minister (Taubira 2012). This includes bans on commercial provision of gametes and the banning of surrogacy.[20] Nonetheless, people do travel from New Caledonia to purchase oocytes in places like the United States (Lévêque 2011) or Spain (interview with IVF practitioner, June 2016).

There are thus diverse forms of mobility from French Polynesia and New Caledonia. The exclusion of same-sex parents from state-supported IVF seems contradictory in the case of French Polynesia where queer parenting and surrogacy are socially acceptable (Zanghellini 2010, 651–77, 2011, 1–30).

CONCLUSIONS

In this chapter we have considered reproductive travel in the Asia-Pacific region, focusing on movements from selected nodal sites—Australia, Japan, and the French Pacific—to disparate destinations. We argue that reproductive travel is inseparable from the processes of globalization, whereby money, products, people, signs, symbols, representations, and practices move (Mackie and Pendleton 2010, n.p.) and that these in turn shape and reorient identities, inequalities, and social relations, as well as complicating the nature and limits of rights. We have provided micro-level case studies which are embedded in an understanding of macro-level global processes (Mackie and Stevens 2009, 269).

We explored the different forms of mobility found in the routes of reproductive travel in the Asia-Pacific region, focusing on techno-scientific mobilities, bodily mobilities, cultural and discursive mobilities, and economic mobilities. We found intersecting routes of reproductive travel, characterized by different degrees of mobility. These movements are shaped by the existence or lack of regulation, gaps between regulatory regimes, gaps between the availability of particular reproductive medical services, the promotion of medical travel and reproductive travel in particular local sites, economic inequality, linguistic or cultural connectedness, historical connections, diasporic connections, postcolonial relationships, and geographical proximity.

These factors come into play in specific local sites and situations. The routes of reproductive travel are not predictable or obvious, but need to be tracked through the kinds of micro-level case studies we have carried out. One site, like Australia, may be a destination for such services as IVF, while Australians travel overseas to access reproductive services not available in their own country. As relatively wealthy countries in the Asia-Pacific region, those from Australia and Japan who travel for reproductive services may move to similar destinations: Thailand and India have, until recently, been destinations for the provision of services unavailable in the commissioning parents' home countries, either because they provided cheaper reproductive labor or because of less stringent laws and regulations.

The US state of Nevada has been a destination because of its clear regulation of matters related to reproductive services, despite the higher costs. Commissioning parents travel to Nevada for clarity on procedures and regulation concerning the provision of third-party gametes, compensated surrogacy, and the naming of commissioning parents on birth certificates (State of Nevada 2007).

Further complexity is illustrated in the case of the French Pacific, where the movements may include those from French Polynesia and New Caledonia toward mainland France, because of its well-developed medical system and medical insurance system. For others, New Zealand may be a destination, where assisted reproduction is available to those outside the heterosexual marriage system. For Indigenous Kanak people, access to IVF is facilitated by financial support to travel to Noumea and by the inclusive attitudes of key staff.

In all three sites, there will be different outcomes when commissioning parents return home. Australia allows for the provision of nationality by descent, while the Japanese courts have so far upheld the principle that the birth mother is the legal mother and her husband is the father. Cross-border reproductive travel by same-sex commissioning parents for surrogacy and/or egg provision is more visible in the Australian context. French laws, currently applied in French Polynesia and New Caledonia, make it difficult for same-sex would-be parents to be open about entering into contracts with gestational mothers or using commercially obtained ova.

The destinations for reproductive travel change with the transformations in regulation in particular sites. Recent controversies in India and Thailand have led to changes in local regulatory regimes, meaning that commissioning parents will seek alternative destinations in the wake of medical practitioners and agents who are constantly on the move in response to changing regulatory conditions. In the French Pacific it was anticipated that the situation could change after the referendum on New Caledonian independence in 2018. In fact, however, the referendum was defeated (Dziedzic and Srinivasan 2018).

The intersections of gender, class, ethnicity, racialized positioning, and relations between the descendants of colonizers and colonized also come into play in shaping "stratified reproduction" (Colen 1995) in "sending" countries. In "destination" countries, too, local regimes of gender, class, ethnicity, racialized positioning, and relations between the descendants of colonizers and colonized come into play in determining which individuals will be the providers of gametes or reproductive labor. India and Thailand were destinations because they had both highly developed reproductive medical industries staffed by élite professionals and poor women who provided gestational services for economic reasons. Some of these providers of gametes or gestational services came from neighboring, even poorer, countries.

What we can learn from these case studies of selected nodal sites in the Asia-Pacific region is that the routes of reproductive travel are shaped by multiple, intersecting, and often contradictory factors. These routes are not easily predictable, but rather must be traced by fine-grained, micro-level local case studies. These case studies also allow us to trace the shifts in the routes of reproductive travel, shaped by changing economic dynamics and changing regulatory regimes. Mobility is thus deeply implicated in the individual, local, and regional politics of reproduction.

NOTES

1. Mattelart (1983); Hannerz (1987, 1989); Giddens (1990); Grewal and Kaplan (1994); Tolentino (1996); and Tambiah (2000).

2. Pande (2011); Inhorn (2011); Hudson et al. (2011); Bergmann (2011a, 2011b); Kroløkke et al. (2012); Crockin (2013); Whittaker and Chee (2016).

3. In April 2016 a West Australian court found that the family had not abandoned Gammy, and allowed the parents to retain custody of Gammy's twin sister (*ABC News* 2016).

4. Mukai (2007); Mackie (2014a); Murdoch (2014); Hawley (2015); Foreign Correspondent (2015).

5. Inhorn and Van Balen (2002); Martin (2009, 2014); Kroløkke and Pant (2012); Crockin (2013); Davies (2017).

6. It was initially hailed as the first birth from a frozen embryo before the 1978 birth in India was properly recognized (Leeton 2013; Kumar 1997).

7. The NHMRC regulates fertility centers in Australia, which need to comply with the appropriate guidelines if they wish to maintain their accreditation.

8. With the recent relaxation of the "one child" policy and the increasing affluence of the middle class in China, Australia has become a destination for IVF treatment, particularly for single Chinese women who could not access such treatment in China (Bolger 2017; see also the Introduction to this volume).

9. Whittaker (2011) argues convincingly that Orientalism underpins views that "family-balancing" by people from countries like Australia is acceptable, whilst sex selection by people from countries like India or China is problematic.

10. http://www.genea.com.au/How-we-can-help/Our-Services/Genetic-Disorders/Sex-selection-with-PGD. Access attempted March 2, 2017, with a Page Not Found response.

11. In Australia, too, small numbers of babies come up for adoption. In Australia, however, there is little stigma attached to being born out of wedlock, with acceptance of de facto marital relationships and around one-third of babies born out of wedlock (Chamie 2017).

12. In June 2013 Sumi Yuki was quoted as having arranged 150 transnational surrogacy agreements resulting in more than 500 births through the provision of ova from third parties. Sumi opened her agency in 1991 (Nishi Nihon Shinbun 2013). Sumi was the agent for the Takadas and introduced them to the Nevada Center for Reproductive Medicine. Information (in Japanese) about the Tokyo center can be seen at Sumiyuki International Limited Company (n.d.).

13. There are two kinds of adoption in Japan. Ordinary adoption (*futsū yōshi engumi*) often involves the adoption of one adult by another. Special adoption (*tokubetsu yōshi engumi*) involves the adoption of a child up to six years old (eight years old where a child has been fostered by the adopting parents); can only be undertaken by a married couple; and usually requires the consent of the relinquishing parents.

14. There are two main ways of determining nationality: jus soli, which depends on the place of birth, and jus sanguinis, which depends on the nationality of the parent(s). Actual practices may, though, take into account a combination of these principles. Jus soli is used in the United States, while jus sanguinis is used in Japan. That is, to acquire Japanese nationality at birth, one needs to have at least one parent of Japanese nationality. Where nationality is not acquired at birth, naturalization is possible in defined circumstances (Mackie 2009).

15. The Takada case followed another case where a couple had been unable to register a child born through a transnational surrogacy agreement.

16. Needless to say, even without using assisted reproduction, there are countless families based on gay or lesbian parenting (Chalmers 2002).

17. Although the main destinations for British people travelling for reproductive services are geographically close locations such as the Czech Republic and Spain, common geographically distant destinations have included the United States, Barbados, India, and South Africa. All of the latter are English-speaking former colonies (Culley et al. 2011), most of which offer cheaper health services.

18. The official numbers are not available on their website (CAFAT n.d.), but according to a presentation by a fertility specialist from the only center in New Caledonia (Caledo Fertilité), up to six IVF cycles are reimbursed at 90 percent (Dechanet et al. undated). This was confirmed in interviews in June 2016 with a range of fertility professionals from New Caledonia.

19. On January 7, 2013, before the vote to legalize same-sex marriage had taken place, an amendment that would have given same-sex couples access to French fertility services was removed. Therefore, same-sex couples, even if married, cannot access France's generous free IVF provisions.

20. In order to discourage people from travelling to access commercial surrogacy, children born in this way were originally not recognized by French law when they returned home (Marvier 2009). This has recently been overturned (Le Conseil D'Etat 2014).

WORKS CITED

AAP. 2015. "New Thai Surrogacy Law Bans Foreigners." *SBS News Australia*. http://www.sbs.com.au/news/article/2015/07/31/new-thai-surrogacy-law-bans-foreigners (Last accessed September 30, 2018).

ABC Background Briefing. 2017. "Surrogacy Secrets." Reporter: Hagar Cohen, February 12. http://www.abc.net.au/radionational/programs/backgroundbriefing/surrogacy-secrets/8252210 (Last accessed September 30, 2018).

ABC News. 2016. "Baby Gammy: Surrogacy Row Family Cleared of Abandoning Child with Down Syndrome in Thailand." April 14. http://www.abc.net.au/news/2016-04-14/baby-gammy-twin-must-remain-with-family-wa-court-rules/7326196 (Last accessed September 30, 2018).

Akersten, M. 2009. "New Caledonia Couple Seeks Baby Joy in NZ." *gaynz.com*, December 10. http://www.gaynz.com/articles/publish/36/article_8288.php (Last accessed September 30, 2018).

Anderson, Warwick. 2009. "From Subjugated Knowledge to Conjugated Subjects: Science and Globalisation, or Postcolonial Studies of Science?" *Postcolonial Studies* 12 (4): 389–400.

———. 2014. "Making Global Health History: The Postcolonial Worldliness of Biomedicine." *Social History of Medicine* 27 (2): 372–84.

Auerbach, Taylor. 2014. "Tiniest Victims of Baby Backlash: Adam and Kate Osborne Stuck in Thailand with their Surrogate Babies Mali and Sierra-Leone." *The Daily Telegraph,* August 19. https://www.dailytelegraph.com.au/news/nsw/tiniest-victims-of-baby-backlash-adam-and-kate-osborne-stuck-in-thailand-with-their-sur rogate-babies-mali-and-sierraleone/news-story/ccc57d87389e5ad61efe9cc4b5299 80e (Last accessed September 3, 2018).

Australian Government Department of Immigration and Border Control. Undated. *Fact Sheet: International Surrogacy Arrangements.* http://www.border.gov.au/about/corporate/information/fact-sheets/36a-surrogacy.

Australian Institute of Health and Welfare. 2012. *Adoptions Australia 2011–12* (Child Welfare Series No. 54). Canberra: Australian Institute of Health and Welfare.

Avril, Pierre and Jean Gicquel. 2013. "Chronique Constitutionnelle Française" [French Constitutional Chronicle]. *Pouvoirs* 3 (146): 171–202.

Bailes, Morry. 2017. "Time to Think of the Children in Surrogacy Cases." *InDaily*, October 26. https://indaily.com.au/opinion/2017/10/26/time-to-think-of-the-children-in-surrogacy-cases/ (Last accessed September 30, 2018).

Barker, Anne. 2017. "'Desperate' Australian Couples Unable to Leave Cambodia with Surrogate Babies." *ABC News.* http://www.abc.net.au/news/2017-02-23/australian-couples-with-surrogate-babies-stuck-in-cambodia/8294810 (Last accessed September 30, 2018).

Barlass, T. 2014. "When Altruistic Surrogacy Goes Wrong." *Sydney Morning Herald*, August 10. http://www.smh.com.au/national/when-altruistic-surrogacy-goes-wrong-20140807-101bo5.html (Last accessed September 30, 2018).

Bastians, Kate. 2016. "'Australian Surrogacy Laws Need to Change': Same Sex Sydney Couple." *Daily Telegraph.* http://www.dailytelegraph.com.au/newslocal/news/australian-surrogacy-laws-need-to-change-sydney-couple/news-story/4ed9845e516b7894d3e353860a822e97 (Last accessed September 30, 2018).

BellyBelly. 2008. "Gender Selection with ICSI." http://www.bellybelly.com.au/forums/long-term-assisted-conception-91/gender-selection-icsi-85971/ (Last accessed March 2, 2017).

Bergmann, Sven. 2011a. "Fertility Tourism: Circumventive Routes That Enable Access to Reproductive Technologies and Substances." *Signs: Journal of Women in Culture and Society* 36 (2): 280–89.

———. 2011b. "Reproductive Agency and Projects: Germans Searching for Egg Donation in Spain and the Czech Republic." *Reproductive Biomedicine Online* 23 (5): 600–8.

Bhangra, Kulraj Singh. 2019. "India's Lower House Passes Bill Banning Commercial Surrogacy." *Bionews* 982 (January 14). Available at https://www.bionews.org.uk/page_140769 (Last accessed February 2, 2019).

Bharadwaj, Aditya. 2002. "Conception Politics: Medical Egos, Media Spotlights, and the Contest over Test-Tube Firsts in India." In *Infertility around the Globe: New Thinking on Childlessness, Gender, and Reproductive Technologies,* edited by Marcia C. Inhorn and Frank Van Balen, 315–33. Berkeley: University of California Press.

Bhowmick, Nilanjana. 2016. "After Nepal, Indian Surrogacy Clinics Move to Cambodia." *Aljazeera.com.* http://www.aljazeera.com/indepth/features/2016/06/nepal-indian-surrogacy-clinics-move-cambodia-160614112517994.html (Last accessed September 30, 2018).

Bolger, Rosemary. 2017. "IVF Tourism: The Chinese Women Travelling to Australia for a Baby." *SBS News.* https://www.sbs.com.au/news/ivf-tourism-the-chinese-women-travelling-to-australia-for-a-baby?cx_cid=edm:newspm:2017 (Last accessed December 30, 2017).

CAFAT. undated. *Régime Unifié d'Assurance Maladie-Maternité* [Unified Health and Maternity Insurance Plan]. https://www.cafat.nc/web/assures/assurance_maladie (Last accessed September 30, 2018).

Chalmers, Sharon. 2002. *Emerging Lesbian Voices from Japan.* London: RoutledgeCurzon.

Chamie, Joseph. 2017. "Out-of-Wedlock Births Rise Worldwide." *Yale Global Online.* https://yaleglobal.yale.edu/content/out-wedlock-births-rise-worldwide (Last accessed December 30, 2017).

Clarke, Adele E., Janet K. Shim, Laura Mamo, Jennifer Ruth Fosket, and Jennifer R. Fishman. 2003. "Biomedicalization: Technoscientific Transformations of Health, Illness, and U.S. Biomedicine." *American Sociological Review* 68 (2): 161–94.

Cohen, Jean, Alan Trounson, Karen Dawson, and Lars Hamberger. 2005. "The Early Days of IVF Outside the UK." *Human Reproduction Update* 11 (5): 439–60.

Colen, Shellee. 1995. "'Like a Mother to Them': Stratified Reproduction and West Indian Childcare Workers and Employers in New York." In *Conceiving the New World Order: The Global Politics of Reproduction*, edited by Faye D. Ginsburg and Rayna Rapp, 78–102. Berkeley: University of California Press.

Commonwealth of Australia. 2016. *Surrogacy Matters: Inquiry into the Regulatory and Legislative Aspects of International and Domestic Surrogacy Arrangements.* Report by the House of Representatives. http://www.aph.gov.au/Parliamentary_Business/Committees/House/Social_Policy_and_Legal_Affairs/Inquiry_into_surrogacy/Report (Last accessed September 9, 2017).

CPS. 2013. *Pendant Votre Grossesse* [During Your Pregnancy]. http://www.cps.pf/espace-assure/droits-et-demarches/par-situation-personnelle/vous-allez-avoir-un-enfant/pendant-votre-grossesse.

Crockin, Susan L. 2013. "Growing Families in a Shrinking World: Legal and Ethical Challenges in Cross-Border Surrogacy." *Reproductive Biomedicine Online* 27 (6): 733–41.

Culley, Lorraine, Nicky Hudson, Frances Rapport, Eric Blyth, Wendy Norton, and Allan A. Pacey. 2011. "Crossing Borders for Fertility Treatment: Motivations, Destinations and Outcomes of UK Fertility Travellers." *Human Reproduction* 26 (9): 2373–81.

Davies, Miranda, ed. 2017. *Babies for Sale?: Transnational Surrogacy, Human Rights and the Politics of Reproduction.* London: Zed Books.

De Castro, Leonardo and Sarah Jane Toledano. 2009. "Bioethics in the Philippines: A Retrospective." *Asian Bioethics Review* 1 (4): 426–44.

De Kretzer, D., P. Dennis, B. Hudson, J. Leeton, A. Lopata, K. Outch, J. Talbot, and C. Wood. 1973. "Transfer of a Human Zygote." *Lancet* 302 (7831): 728–29.

Dechanet, Clothilde, Patrick Hiltenbrand, Nathalie Colas, and Erick Camus. n.d. *Assistance Médicale à la Procréation (AMP) en Nouvelle Caledonie* [Medically Assisted Reproduction (MAR) in New Caledonia]. http://www.cht.nc/doc/JMC%20sur%20internet/Laperouse/Assistance%20M%C3%A9dicale%20%C3%A0%20la%20Procr%C3%A9ation.pdf (Last accessed September 30, 2018).

Deomampo, Daisy. 2013. "Gendered Geographies of Reproductive Tourism." *Gender & Society* 27 (4): 514–37.

Dey, Sushmi. 2018. "Lok Sabha Clears Bill Banning Commercial Surrogacy." *Times of India*, December 20. Available at https://timesofindia.indiatimes.com/india/lok-sabha-passes-surrogacy-regulation-bill-2016-which-bans-commercial-surrogacy/articleshow/67165408.cms (Last accessed February 2, 2019).

Dimoia, John. 2013. "Blastocysts and Family Planning: IVF and Tracking a Developmental Context for Biomedical Research in Singapore (1966–1994)." *Science Technology & Society* 18 (3): 275–89.

Dobbin, Marika. 2016. "IVF Treatment: South African Agency Flies Egg Donors to Australia." *Sydney Morning Herald*, February 8. http://www.smh.com.au/national/ivf-treatment-south-african-agency-flies-egg-donors-to-australia-20160208-gmo8qn.html (Last accessed September 30, 2018).

Dorney, Sean. 2013. "New Caledonia Struggles with High Cost of Living." *ABC News*, July 10, 2013. http://www.abc.net.au/news/2013-07-10/an-new-caledonia-struggles-with-high-cost-of-living/4810870 (Last accessed September 30, 2018).

Dziedzic, Stephen and Prianka Srinivasan. 2018. "New Caledonia Narrowly Rejects Independence from France in Historic Referendum." *ABC News*, November 5, 2018. https://www.abc.net.au/news/2018-11-05/new-caledonia-rejects-independence-from-france/10464248 (Last accessed June 14, 2019).

Eschle, Catherine. 2002. "Engendering Global Democracy." *International Feminist Journal of Politics* 4 (3): 315–41.

Everingham, Sam. 2014. "Use of Surrogacy by Australians: Implications for Policy and Law Reform." In *Families, Policy and the Law: Selected Essays on Contemporary Issues for Australia*, edited by Australian Institute of Family Studies, 67–79. Canberra: Australian Institue of Family Studies.

Fan, Fa-Ti. 2012. "The Global Turn in the History of Science." *East Asian Science, Technology and Society* 6 (2): 249–58.

Fertility Associates. 2014. *Chemin vers un Enfant* [Journey towards a Child]. http://www.fertilityassociates.co.nz/francais/Chemin-Vers-Un-Enfant.aspx.

Fertility Society of Australia. 2013. "New Data Reveals Growing Trend in Australian Couples Seeking Social Sex Selection in Overseas IVF Units." September 2. www.fertilitysociety.com.au/wp-content/uploads/Bowman-Social-Sex-Selection_.doc (Last accessed September 30, 2018).

Fivfrance.com. 2014. *AMP: Coûts et Remboursements Autorisés en France en 2014* MAR [Medically Assisted Reproduction: Authorized Costs and Reimbursements in France in 2014]. http://www.fivfrance.com/page_quest06.html (Last accessed September 30, 2018).

Foreign Correspondent (Australian Broadcasting Corporation). 2014. "The Baby Makers: Critics Push for Regulation of India's Booming Surrogacy Industry." *ABC News*, August 5. http://www.abc.net.au/news/2014-04-15/babymakers-critics-push-for-regulation-india-surrogacy/5389678 (Last accessed September 30, 2018).

———. 2015. "India Surrogacy Case: Documents Show New South Wales Couple Abandoned Baby Boy Despite Warnings." *ABC News*, April 13. http://www.abc.

net.au/news/2015-04-13/australian-couple-abandon-baby-boy-in-india-surrogacy-case/6387206 (Last accessed September 30, 2018).

Forum de Fiv.fr. 2017. *FIV en Nouvelle-Zélande* [IVF in New Zealand]. October 13. https://forum.fiv.fr/viewtopic.php?t=5124 (Last accessed September 30, 2018).

Forum Naissance en Polynésie. 2012. *Remboursement CPS des FIV* [CPS [Polynesian Social Security Fund] IVF Reimbursements]. http://bbfenua.frbb.net/t12-remboursement-cps-des-fiv (Last accessed September 30, 2018).

Four Corners (Australian Broadcasting Corporation). 2016. "The Baby Business." May 31. http://www.abc.net.au/4corners/stories/2016/05/30/4469652.htm (Last accessed September 30, 2018).

Franklin, Sarah. 2007. "'Crook' Pipettes: Embryonic Emigrations from Agriculture to Reproductive Biomedicine." *Studies in History and Philosophy of Science Part C: Studies in History and Philosophy of Biological and Biomedical Sciences* 38 (2): 358–73.

———. 2013. *Biological Relatives: IVF, Stem Cells, and the Future of Kinship*. Durham: Duke University Press.

Genea. 2013. *Sex Selection*. http://www.genea.com.au/my-fertility/i-need-help/fertility-treatments/sex-selection.

Giddens, Anthony. 1990. *The Consequences of Modernity*. Cambridge: Polity.

Google Baby. 2009. Directed by Zippi Brand Frank. Distributed by Films Transit International.

Government of India. 2018. The Surrogacy Regulation Bill, Bill No 257-C of 2016, Passed by Lok Sabha on December 19, 2018.

Government of Thailand. 2015. Protection for Children Born through Assisted Reproductive Technologies Act, BE 2558, Enacted February 19, 2015.

Grewal, Inderpal and Caren Kaplan. 1994. *Scattered Hegemonies: Postmodernity and Transnational Feminist Practices*. Minneapolis: University of Minnesota Press.

Hannerz, Ulf. 1987. "The World in Creolization." *Africa* 57 (4): 546–49.

———. 1989. "Notes on the Global Ecumene." *Public Culture* 1 (2): 66–75.

Hawley, Samantha. 2015. "Baby Gammy, One Year Old at Centre of Thai Surrogacy Scandal, Granted Australian Citizenship." *ABC News*, January 20. http://www.abc.net.au/news/2015-01-20/baby-gammy-granted-australian-citizenship/6026600 (Last accessed September 30, 2018).

Hudson, Nicky, Lorraine Culley, Eric Blyth, and Allan Pacey. 2011. "Cross-Border Reproductive Care: A Review of the Literature." *Reproductive Biomedicine Online* 22 (7): 673–85.

Inhorn, Marcia C. 2011. "Diasporic Dreaming: Return Reproductive Tourism to the Middle East." *Reproductive Biomedicine Online* 23 (5): 582–91.

Inhorn, Marcia C. and Frank Van Balen, eds. 2002. *Infertility around the Globe: New Thinking on Childlessness, Gender, and Reproductive Technologies*. Berkeley: University of California Press.

Ishii, Michiko. 2009. "Medically Assisted Reproduction and Family Law in Japan." In *Japanese Family Law in Comparative Perspective*, edited by Harry Scheiber and Laurent Mayali, 175–201. Berkeley: Robbins Collection.

IVF Australia. n.d. *International Patients.* http://www.ivf.com.au/international-patients (Last accessed September 30, 2018).

Japan Times. 2015. "Thai Surrogates, Japanese Dad Try to Reclaim Babies." January 15. http://www.japantimes.co.jp/news/2015/01/15/national/thai-surrogate-mothers-seek-court-order-reclaim-babies/#.VVVJtVaOWlI (Last accessed September 30, 2018).

Johnson, Martin H. 2006. "Escaping the Tyranny of the Embryo? A New Approach to ART Regulation Based on UK and Australian Experiences." *Human Reproduction* 21 (11): 2756–65.

Kahn, Susan Martha. 2002. "Rabbis and Reproduction: The Uses of New Reproductive Technologies among Ultraorthodox Jews in Israel." In *Infertility around the Globe: New Thinking on Childlessness, Gender, and Reproductive Technologies,* edited by Marcia C. Inhorn and Frank Van Balen, 283–97. Berkeley: University of California Press.

Kamin, Debra. 2015. "Israel Evacuates Surrogate Babies From Nepal but Leaves the Mothers Behind." April 28, 2015. http://time.com/3838319/israel-nepal-surrogates/ (Last accessed September 30, 2018).

Kinjō, Kiyoko. 1996. *Seishoku Kakumei to Jinken: Umu koto ni jiyū wa aru no ka* [The Reproductive Revolution and Human Rights: Is there Freedom in Bearing Children?]. Tokyo: Chūkō Shinsho.

Kroløkke, Charlotte Halmø and Saumya Pant. 2012. "'I Only Need Her Uterus': Neo-Liberal Discourses on Transnational Surrogacy." *NORA: Nordic Journal of Feminist and Gender Research* 20 (4): 233–48.

Kroløkke, Charlotte Halmø, Karen A. Foss, and Saumya Pant. 2012. "Fertility Travel: The Commodification of Human Reproduction: Charlotte Kroløkke, Karen A. Foss, and Saumya Pant, Guest Editors." *Cultural Politics* 8 (2): 273–82.

Kumar, T. C. Anand. 1997. "Architect of India's First Test Tube Baby: Dr Subhas Mukerji, 16 January 1931 to 19 July 1981." *Current Science* 72 (7): 526–31.

Kyodo News. 2018. "Thai Court Gives Japanese Man Custody of 13 Surrogate Children." February 20. https://english.kyodonews.net/news/2018/02/00d9b6a10ced-thai-court-gives-japanese-man-custody-of-13-surrogate-children.html (Last accessed September 30, 2018).

Lateline (Australian Broadcasting Corporation). 2017. "Women Using IVF to Choose the Sex of Their Children Break Silence on 'Gender Disappointment.'" *ABC News,* February 7. http://www.abc.net.au/news/2017-02-07/women-using-ivf-to-choose-sex-of-their-babies/8234798 (Last accessed September 30, 2018).

Le Conseil d'Etat. 2014. *Gestation pour Autrui (GPA)* [Gestational Surrogacy]. Décembre 12, 2014. http://www.conseil-etat.fr/Actualites/Communiques/Gestation-pour-autrui-GPA?utm_campaign=cp&utm_medium=circ&utm_source=twt (Last accessed September 30, 2018).

Le Forum de FIV.Fr. 2014. *FIV ICSI avec DPI* [IVF ICSI with PGD [IVF Intra-Cytoplasmic Sperm Injection with Pre-Implantation Genetic Diagnosis]]. http://forum.fiv.fr/fiv-et-pma-f3/fiv-icsi-avec-dpi-t608-12.html (Last accessed September 30, 2018).

Leeton, John. 2004. "The Early History of IVF in Australia and its Contribution to the World (1970–1990)." *Australian New Zealand Journal of Obstetrics and Gynaecology* 44 (6): 495–501.

———. 2013. *Test Tube Revolution: The Early History of IVF*. Clayton: Monash University Publishing.

Les Nouvelles Calédoniennes. 2005. "Fécondation in Vitro: NYLS Ouvre la Voie de l'Espoir" [In Vitro Fertilisation: NYLS Opens the Door to Hope]. March 14. http://www.lnc.nc/article/societe/fecondation-in-vitro-nyls-ouvre-la-voie-de-l-espoir (Last accessed September 30, 2018).

Löwy, Ilana. 2006. "La Fabrication du Naturel: L'Assistance Médicale à la Procréation dans une Perspective Comparée" [Making the Natural: Medically Assisted Reproduction in Comparative Perspective]. *Tumultes* 1 (26): 35–55.

Mackie, Vera. 2009. "Family Law and its Others." In *Japanese Family Law in Comparative Perspective*, edited by Harry Scheiber and Laurent Mayali, 139–63. Berkeley: Robbins Collection.

———. 2013. "Genders and Genetics: The Legal and Medical Regulation of Family Forms in Japan." *Australian Journal of Asian Law* 14 (1): 1–18.

———. 2014a. "Birth Registration and the Right to Have Rights: The Changing Family and the Unchanging Koseki." In *Japan's Household Registration System and Citizenship: Koseki, Identification and Documentation,* edited by David Chapman and Karl J. Krogness, 203–20. London: Routledge.

———. 2014b. "Science, Society and the Sea of Fertility: New Reproductive Technologies in Japanese Popular Culture." *Japan Forum* 26 (4): 441–61.

Mackie, Vera and Carolyn S. Stevens. 2009. "Globalisation and Body Politics." *Asian Studies Review* 33 (3): 257–73.

Mackie, Vera and Mark Pendleton. 2010. "On the Move: Globalisation and Culture in the Asia-Pacific Region." *Intersections: Gender, History and Culture in the Asian Context* 23: 1–11.

Martin, Lauren Jade. 2009. "Reproductive Tourism in the Age of Globalization." *Globalizations* 6 (2): 249–63.

———. 2014. "The World's Not Ready for This: Globalizing Selective Technologies." *Science, Technology, & Human Values* 39 (3): 432–55.

Marvier, Marie. 2009. "Mère Porteuse - Témoignage: 'Officiellement, Nos Filles n'ont Pas de Mère'" [Gestational Mothers—Testimony: Officially, Our Daughters do not Have a Mother]. *France Soir*, June 22. http://archive.francesoir.fr/pratique/sante/mere-porteuse-temoignage-%E2%80%9Cofficiellement-nos-filles-n%E2%80%99ont-pas-mere%E2%80%9D-39690.html (Last accessed September 30, 2018).

Mattelart, Armand. 1983. *Transnationals and the Third World: The Struggle for Culture*. Trans. D. Buxton. South Hadley, MA: Bergin and Garvey Publishers.

Medibridge. undated. http://www.medi-bridges.com/ (Last accessed September 30, 2018).

Merle, Isabelle. 2000. "De l'Idée de Cantonnement à la Constitution des Réserves: La Définition de la Proprieté Indigène" [From the Idea of Cantonization o the Creation of Reservations: The Definition of Indigenous Property]. In *En Pays Kanak;*

Ethnology, Linguistique Archéology, Histoire de la Nouvelle Calédonie, edited by Alban Bensa and Isabelle Leblic, 217–34. Paris: Maison des Sciences de l'Homme.
Millbank, Jenni. 2012. "From Alice and Evelyn to Isabella: Exploring the Narratives and Norms of 'New' Surrogacy in Australia." *Griffith Law Review* 21 (1): 101–36.
Miller, Barbara. 2012. "From Here to Maternity." *Sydney Morning Herald*, December 22. http://www.smh.com.au/lifestyle/from-here-to-maternity-20121218-2bl9d.html (Last accessed September 30, 2018).
———. 2017. "Women using IVF to Choose the Sex of Their Children Break Silence on 'Gender Disappointment.'" *ABC News Online*, February 17. http://www.abc.net.au/news/2017-02-07/women-using-ivf-to-choose-sex-of-their-babies/8234798 (Last accessed September 30, 2018).
Ministère des Outre-Mer. n.d. *Découvrir Les Outre-Mer* [Discovering the Overseas [Territories and Countries]]. http://www.outre-mer.gouv.fr/?-decouvrir-l-outre-mer-.html (Last accessed September 30, 2018).
Monash IVF. 2012. *The History of IVF: A Chronology*. http://monashivf.com/the-history-of-ivf-a-chronology/ (Last accessed September 30, 2018).
Mukai, Aki. 2002a [2001]. *16shū: Anata to Ita Shiawasena Jikan* [16 Weeks: Happy Times with You]. Tokyo: Fusōsha.
———. 2002b. *Aitakatta: Dairibo Shussan to iu Sentaku* [I Wanted to Meet You: The Choice of Surrogate Birth]. Tokyo: Gentōsha.
———. 2004. *Puropōzu: Watashitachi no Kodomo o Unde Kudasai* [Proposal: Please Bear Our Child]. Tokyo: Magajin Hausu.
———. 2007. *Kazoku Miman* [Not Quite a Family]. Tokyo: Shōgakukan.
Murdoch, Lindsay. 2014. "Crackdown on Thailand Surrogacy Industry Puts Australian Couples in Limbo." *Sydney Morning Herald*, August 11. http://www.smh.com.au/world/crackdown-on-thailand-surrogacy-industry-puts-australian-couples-in-limbo-20140811-102se9.html (Last accessed September 30, 2018).
———. 2017. "A Mother's Anguish as Gammy Celebrates Fourth Birthday." *Stuff*, December 24. https://www.stuff.co.nz/life-style/parenting/100156066/a-mothers-anguish-as-gammy-celebrates-fourth-birthday (Last accessed September 30, 2018).
Natisens. n.d. *Sécurité Sociale et PMA* [Social Security and MAR [Medically Assisted Reproduction]]. http://www.natisens.com/Articles/Administration/Secu_France.html (Last accessed September 30, 2018).
Netsu, Yahiro and Sawami Ryōko. 2009. *Haha to Musume no Dairi Shussan* [Mother and Daughter Surrogate Birth]. Tokyo: Haru Shobō.
Nishi Nihon Shunbun. 2013. "Konnichi wa akachan dai rokubu: Kōdo Seishoku Iryō wa Ima 2 Dairi Shussan Risuku Kangaete" [Hello Baby Part Six: The Current State of High Level Reproductive Medicine 2 Thinking of the Risks of Surrogate Birth]. June 18. http://www.nishinippon.co.jp/feature/life_topics/article/20923 (Last accessed September 30, 2018).
Noda, Seiko and Yahiro Netsu. 2011. *Kono Kuni de Umu to iu koto* [To Bear Children in this Country]. Tokyo: Popura-sha.
Pande, Amrita. 2010. "Commercial Surrogacy in India: Manufacturing a Perfect Mother-Worker." *Signs* 35 (4): 969–92.
———. 2011. "Transnational Commercial Surrogacy in India: Gifts for Global Sisters?" *Reproductive Biomedicine Online* 23 (5): 618–25.

———. 2017. "Gestational Surrogacy in India: New Dynamics of Reproductive Labour." In *Critical Perspectives on Work and Employment in Globalizing India*, edited by Ernesto Noronha and Premilla D'Cruz, 267–82. Singapore: Springer Singapore.

Points, Kari. n.d. *Commercial Surrogacy and Fertility Tourism in India: The Case of Baby Manji*. Durham: The Kenan Institute for Ethics at Duke University. https://kenan.ethics.duke.edu/wp-content/uploads/2012/08/BabyManji_TN2015.pdf.

Report Buyer. 2016. *Asia Pacific Infertility (Testing And Treatment) Market Forecast 2016–2022*. https://www.reportbuyer.com/product/4461526/asia-pacific-infertility-testing-and-treatment-market-forecast-2016-2022.html (Last accessed September 30, 2018).

Ringler, Guy. 2016. "A California Doctor is Helping Build Gay Families in Japan." *Advocate*, January 6. https://www.advocate.com/commentary/2016/1/06/california-doctor-helping-build-gay-families-japan (Last accessed September 30, 2018).

Ris, Catherine. 2013. "Les Inégalités Ethniques dans l'Accès à l'Emploi en Nouvelle-Calédonie" [Ethnic Inequalities in Employment Access in New Caledonia]. *Economie et Statistique* 464–465–466: 59–72.

Rodino, Iolanda S., Sonja Goedeke, and Sarah Nowoweiski. 2014. "Motivations and Experiences of Patients Seeking Cross-Border Reproductive Care: The Australian and New Zealand Context." *Fertility and Sterility* 102 (5): 1422–31.

Roubio Collet, Nathalie. 2012. "Comparaison des Prix entre la Nouvelle-Calédonie et la Métropole" [Price Comparison between New Caledonia and the Metropolis]. *Les Synthèses de CEROM*. http://www.cerom-outremer.fr/IMG/pdf/cerom_-_comparaison_prix_entre_nc_et_metropole_-_octobre_2012.pdf (Last accessed September 30, 2018).

SBS News. 2015. "New Thai Surrogacy Law Bans Foreigners." July 31. http://www.sbs.com.au/news/article/2015/07/31/new-thai-surrogacy-law-bans-foreigners (Last accessed September 30, 2018).

Science Council of Japan, Assisted Reproductive Technologies Review Committee. 2008. *Issues Related to the Assisted Reproductive Technologies Centered on Surrogate Pregnancy: Toward a Social Consensus*. http://www.scj.go.jp/ja/info/kohyo/pdf/kohyo-20-t56-1e.pdf (Last accessed September 30, 2018).

Semba, Yukari, Chungfang Chang, Hyunsoo Hong, Ayako Kamisato, Minori Kokado, and Kaori Muto. 2010. "Surrogacy: Donor Conception Regulation in Japan." *Bioethics* 24 (7): 348–57.

Shalev, Carmel, Hedva Eyal, and Etti Samama. 2017. "Transnational Surrogacy and the Earthquake in Nepal: A Case Study from Israel." In *Babies for Sale?: Transnational Surrogacy, Human Rights and the Politics of Reproduction*, edited by Miranda Davies, 49–64. London: Zed Books.

Spar, Debora. 2007. "The Egg Trade: Making Sense of the Market for Human Oocytes." *New England Journal of Medicine* 356 (13): 1289–91.

Spooner, Rania and Broede Carmody. 2016. "'Madness' AMA President Says Woman having Baby at 62 is 'Selfish and Wrong.'" *Sydney Morning Herald*, August 3. http://www.smh.com.au/national/madness--ama-president-says-woman-havin

g-baby-at-62-is-selfish-and-wrong-20160803-gqjt8f.html (Last accessed 30 September 2018).
State of Nevada. 2007. Nevada Revised Statutes. Chapter 126.
Steptoe, Patrick C. and Robert G. Edwards. 1978. "Successful Birth after IVF." *Lancet* 312: 366.
Stockey-Bridge, Michaela. 2018. *The Lure of Hope: On the Transnational Surrogacy Trail from Australia to India.* Vancouver: Fairleigh Dickinson University Press.
Stokes, Katrina. 2015. "SA Fertility Clinic to Import Donor Eggs from America Because of Growing Demand." *The Advertiser*, January 19. http://www.adelaidenow.com.au/news/south-australia/sa-fertility-clinic-to-import-donor-eggs-from-america-because-of-growing-demand/news-story/44f7731f343f23cf061273a2f51206b1 (Last accessed September 30, 2018).
Sumiyuki International Limited Company. undated. *Ranshi Teikyō* [Provision of Ova]. *Dairibo Shussan Jōhō Sentā* [Surrogate Birth Information Center]. http://www.sumiyuki.co.jp/index.html (Last accessed September 30, 2018).
Superior ART. 2007. *About Superior A.R.T.* http://www.thaisuperiorart.com/about.php (Last accessed March 2, 2017).
Suzuki, Masakuni. 2014. "In Vitro Fertilization in Japan: Early Days of in Vitro Fertilization and Embryo Transfer and Future Prospects for Assisted Reproductive Technology." *Proceedings of the Japan Academy, Series B, Physical and Biological Sciences* 90 (5): 184–201.
Tambiah, Stanley J. 2000. "Transnational Movements, Diaspora and Multiple Modernities." *Daedalus* 129: 163–94.
Taubira, Christiane. 2012. "Gestation Pour Autrui (GPA)" [Gestational Surrogacy]. *Archives Lu Vu Entendu*, November 7. http://www.presse.justice.gouv.fr/lu-vu-entendu-11603/archives-lu-vu-entendu-de-2012-12422/gestation-pour-autrui-gpa-24764.html (Last accessed September 30, 2018).
Tolentino, Roland B. 1996. "Bodies, Letters, Catalogues: Filipinas in Transnational Space." *Social Text* 14 (3): 49–76.
United Nations. 2015. *Non-Self-Governing Territories.* http://www.un.org/en/decolonization/nonselfgovterritories.shtml (Last accessed September 30, 2018).
Wamytan, Roch. 2005. "New Caledonia Still a Colony Despite Accord." *Pacific Island Report*, unpaginated, October 27. http://archives.pireport.org/archive/2005/October/10-27-com.htm (Last accessed September 30, 2018).
Wasmer, Etienne and Quentin David. 2012. "Rapport sur la Situation Economique de la Nouvelle-Calédonie: Et si la Prospérité n'Etait pas Eternelle?" [Report on New Caledonia's Economic Situation: What if Prosperity wasn't Forever?]. *UFC Que Choisir Nouvelle Calédonie*, August. http://www.ufcnouvellecaledonie.nc/wp-content/uploads/2013/12/situation-economique-de-la-nc.pdf (Last accessed September 30, 2018).
Whittaker, Andrea. 2009. "Global Technologies and Transnational Reproduction in Thailand." *Asian Studies Review* 33 (3): 319–32.
———. 2011. "Reproduction Opportunists in the New Global Sex Trade: PGD and Non-Medical Sex Selection." *Reproductive Biomedicine Online* 23 (5): 609–17.

———. 2016. “From ‘Mung Ming’ to ‘Baby Gammy’: A Local History of Assisted Reproduction in Thailand.” *Reproductive Biomedicine & Society Online* 2: 71–78.

———. 2016b. “Circumvention, Crisis and Confusion: Australians Crossing Borders to Thailand for International Surrogacy.” In *Assisted Reproductive Technologies in the Global South and North: Issues, Challenges and the Future*, edited by Virginie Rozée and Sayeed Unisa, 113–127. Oxford: Routledge.

———. 2018. *International Surrogacy as Disruptive Industry in Southeast Asia*. New Brunswick: Rutgers University Press.

Whittaker, Andrea and Amy Speier. 2010. “‘Cycling Overseas’: Care, Commodification, and Stratification in Cross-Border Reproductive Travel.” *Medical Anthropology* 29 (4): 363–83.

Whittaker, Andrea and Heng Leng Chee. 2016. “‘Flexible Bio-Citizenship’ and International Medical Travel: Transnational Mobilities for Care in Asia.” *International Sociology* 31 (3): 286–304.

Wood, Anthony. 2015. “Surrogacy: A Personal Perspective.” In *Surrogacy, Law and Human Rights*, edited by Paula Gerber and Katie Byrne, 9–12. London: Routledge.

Wu, Chia-Ling. 2012. “IVF Policy and Global/Local Politics: The Making of Multiple-Embryo Transfer Regulation in Taiwan.” *Social Science & Medicine* 75 (4): 725–32.

Zanghellini, Aleardo. 2010. “Queer Kinship Practices in Non-Western Contexts: French Polynesia’s Gender-Variant Parents and the Law of La République.” *Journal of Law and Society* 37 (4): 651–77.

———. 2011. “Gay Surrogacy, Intentionality and Tahitian Parenting.” *Griffith Law Review* 20 (1): 1–30.

Zocca, Franco. 2006. “New Caledonia.” In *Globalization and the Re-Shaping of Christianity in the Pacific Islands,* edited by Manfred Ernst, 265–316. Suva: The Pacific Theological College.

Index

About the Contributors

Sarah Ferber is a cultural historian, who researches European religious history and modern medical history. Her books include *Bioethics in Historical Perspective* (Palgrave 2013) and *The Body Divided* (Ashgate 2012, co-edited with Sally Wilde). She is Honorary Professorial Fellow in the History Program, University of Wollongong.

Vera Mackie is senior professor of Asian and international studies and director of the Centre for Critical Human Rights Research in the Faculty of Law, Humanities and the Arts at the University of Wollongong. Recent publications include *Remembering Women's Activism* (2019, coauthored with Sharon Crozier-De Rosa); *The Social Sciences in the Asian Century* (2015, coedited with Carol Johnson and Tessa Morris-Suzuki); *Ways of Knowing about Human Rights in Asia* (2015); *The Routledge Handbook of Sexuality Studies in East Asia* (2015, coedited with Mark McLelland); and *Gender, Nation and State in Modern Japan* (2014, coedited with Andrea Germer and Ulrike Wöhr).

Nicola J. Marks is senior lecturer in sociology in the Faculty of Law, Humanities and the Arts at the University of Wollongong. She has a background in human genetics (University of Cambridge) and science and technology studies (University of Edinburgh). She researches and lectures in the social dimensions of health and medicine. She has published on public engagement in science, the social construction of stem cell research, and discourse analysis in journals such as *Public Understanding of Science*, *New Genetics and Society*, and *Sociological Review*. She is vice president of the Australasian Association for the History, Philosophy and Social Studies of

Science, and a member of the National Committee for History and Philosophy of Science (Australian Academy of Sciences).

Jane Adams is a medico-legal historian, whose research centers on the intersections between law, medicine, fertility, and family formation. She completed her PhD on New Zealand's modern history of infertility and assisted reproductive technologies in 2017. She was then a postdoctoral fellow with the University of Otago Legal Issues Centre, researching historical issues about access to justice and legal architecture. Jane currently lectures in New Zealand history topics in the History Programme at the University of Otago, Dunedin, New Zealand.

Sarah Franklin is a social scientist who has published extensively on the social implications of new reproductive technologies, and in particular the changing status of the biological, since the 1980s. Her books include *Embodied Progress* (1997), *Born and Made* (2006), *Dolly Mixtures* (2007), and *Biological Relatives* (2013). She is the founding director of the Reproductive Sociology Research Group (ReproSoc) and leads the British Academy–funded IVF Histories and Cultures Project at the University of Cambridge, where she was elected to the Chair of Sociology in 2011. Franklin is coeditor in chief, with Professor Martin Johnson, of the journal *Reproductive Biomedicine and Society* and codirects the Wellcome Trust–funded project Changing (In)Fertilities, with Dr. Marcia Inhorn.

Jaya Keaney completed her PhD in the Department of Gender and Cultural Studies at the University of Sydney in 2019. Her PhD explores ontologies of race in queer families who conceive children through reproductive technologies, employing interview methods. Jaya was a visiting scholar with the Reproductive Technologies Research Group (Reprosoc) at the University of Cambridge in 2018. Her broader research interests include feminist science studies, affect theory, sensory ethnography and queer of colour critique.

Vasudha Mohanka is a PhD candidate in the School of Humanities and Social Inquiry at the University of Wollongong in Australia. Her PhD is funded by the Australian Research Council Discovery Project "IVF and Assisted Reproduction: The Global Experience." Vasudha's dissertation outlines the history of human in vitro fertilization in India, analyzing language and metaphors in a popularly circulated, fortnightly English news magazine in India since 1978. Her primary research interests are feminist phenomenology, (dis)embodiment, feminist science studies, precarity, eugenics, reproductive technologies, and affect.

Robyn Morris, PhD, is based at the University of Wollongong, Australia. Her areas of interest include diaspora studies, trauma and memory studies, and the politics of citizenship and belonging. Her focus is trauma narratives in diasporic Asian writing. She has published widely on the works of writers such as Larissa Lai, Joy Kogawa, Hiromi Goto, Evelyn Lau, Lillian Ng, Simone Lazaroo, Hsu-Ming Teo, Madeleine Thien, and Alice Pung in articles, book chapters, interviews, and reviews. She is the editor of *Australasian Canadian Studies* and president of the Association for Canadian Studies in Australia and New Zealand (ACSANZ).

Damien W. Riggs is a professor in psychology at Flinders University and an Australian Research Council Future Fellow. He is the author of over 200 publications in the areas of family, gender, and mental health, including *Working with Transgender Young People and Their Families: A Critical Developmental Approach* (Palgrave, 2019).

Sonja van Wichelen is an associate professor in the Department of Sociology and Social Policy at the University of Sydney. Her current project (funded by a Discovery Early Career Researcher Award from the Australian Research Council) investigates the impact of globalization and biomedicine on the legal governance of family life. She is the author of *Legitimating Life: Adoption in the Age of Globalization and Biotechnology* (2018) and *Religion, Gender and Politics in Indonesia: Disputing the Muslim Body* (2010), and coeditor of *Commitment and Complicity in Cultural Theory and Practice* (2009). Together with Marc de Leeuw she is editor of the new book series *Biolegalities* and is preparing a manuscript with the provisional title *Biolegalities: A Critical Intervention.*

Andrea Whittaker is a former ARC Future Fellow in anthropology in the School of Social Sciences at Monash Univeristy. Her current research projects include the study of global medical trade and mobility, reproductive travel and biotechnologies in the Asia-Pacific, including issues of gender, religion, bioethics, and global regulation of the trade, and social isolation among HIV positive people in Queensland. Her publications include *International Surrogacy as Disruptive Technology in South East Asia* (2019); Thai *In Vitro: Assisted reproductive technologies in Thailand* (2015); *Abortion, Sin and the State in Thailand* (2004), and *Intimate Knowledge: Women and Their Health in Northeast Thailand* (2000).